The Little Black Book of Geriatrics

Karen Gershman, MD, CMD, CAQ Geriatrics

Professor of Community and Family Medicine
Dartmouth Medical School

Faculty, Maine-Dartmouth Family Practice Residency Program
Augusta, Maine

Dennis M. McCullough, MD, CAQ Geriatrics

Medical Director, Kendal at Hanover
Hanover, New Hampshire

Associate Professor and Chief Clinical Officer
Department of Community and Family Medicine
Dartmouth-Hitchcock Medical Center
Lebanon, New Hampshire

General Series Editor

Daniel K. Onion, MD, MPH, FACP
Professor of Community and Family Medicine
Dartmouth Medical School
Hanover, New Hampshire

Director, Maine-Dartmouth Family Practice Residency Program
Augusta, Maine

Other titles in the series:

Onion: The Little Black Book of Primary Care, 2nd edition

Blackwell
Science

© 1998 by Blackwell Science, Inc.
Editorial offices:
350 Main Street, Malden, MA 02148-5018, USA
Osney Mead, Oxford OX2 0EL, England
25 John Street, London WC1N 2BL, England
23 Ainslie Place, Edinburgh EH3 6AJ, Scotland
54 University Street, Carlton, Victoria 3053, Australia

Other editorial offices:
Blackwell Wissenschafts-Verlag GmbH
Kurfürstendamm 57
10707 Berlin, Germany

Blackwell Science KK
MG Kodenmacho Building
7–10 Kodenmacho Nihombashi
Chuo-ku, Tokyo 104, Japan

First published 1998

Acquisitions: Joy Denomme
Production: Karen Feeney
Manufacturing: Lisa Flanagan
Typeset by Achorn Graphic Services, Inc.
Printed and bound by Edwards Brothers

Printed in the United States of America
98 99 00 01 5 4 3 2

The Blackwell Science logo is a trade mark of Blackwell Science Ltd, registered at the United Kingdom Trade Marks Registry.

Distributors:
Marston Book Services Ltd
PO Box 269
Abingdon, Oxon OX14 4YN, England
(*Orders:* Tel: 44-01235-465500
            Fax: 44-01235-465555)

USA
Blackwell Science, Inc.
Commerce Place
350 Main Street
Malden, MA 02148-5018
(*Orders:* Tel: 800-759-6102
            617-388-8250
            Fax: 617-388-8255)

Canada
Copp Clark Professional
200 Adelaide Street, West, 3rd Floor
Toronto, Ontario M5H 1W7
(*Orders:* Tel: 800-815-9417
            416-597-1616
            Fax: 416-597-1617)

Australia
Blackwell Science Pty Ltd
54 University Street
Carlton, Victoria 3053
(*Orders:* Tel: 3-9347-0300
            Fax: 3-9349-3016)

Library of Congress Cataloging-in-Publication Data
Gershman, Karen.
   The little black book of geriatrics / Karen Gershman, Dennis M. McCollough.
      p. cm.
      Includes bibliographical references.
      ISBN 0-632-04328-8
      1. Geriatrics—Handbooks, manuals, etc. I. McCullough, Dennis M. II. Title.
      [DNLM: 1. Geriatrics—handbooks. WT 39 G381L 1997]
RC952.55.G485   1997
618.97—dc21
DNLM/DLC
for Library of Congress   97-37996
                                CIP

Contents

To Miriam Axelrod, MD and Melaine Gershman-Tewksbury, MD, who in kindling hope in their patients have given off a great light.

To my father, who thought I should be a physician, and to my mother and father whose excellent examples as teachers inspired me to be both.

K.G.

To Pamela Harrison, poet and partner, and our daughter Kate, who have always graciously supported my professional and personal journeys.

D.M.

Preface

In college, I had the habit of reading good literature in the bathtub, late at night, sometimes until 2 or 3 in the morning. As my eyelids and hands went limp, lulled by the warm water and slumber, the book would inevitably tumble. Now, most of my treasured library is a bit waterlogged, the pages bunched and wrinkled after hanging to dry.

I could attribute my novels' misadventures to my father, a professor of microbiology. It was he who insisted that the dreaded sciences: organic chemistry, comparative physiology, physics, be tackled early in the evening. "Save the humanities for later." My precious humanities were like dessert. They accompanied the reward of a tepid tub after an arduous day of classes.

In Herman Hesse's *The Glass Bead Game,* the main character of the book, the aged and esteemed master of the glass bead game, has taken on a young apprentice. The student is unfocused, inexperienced, and restless, yet the sage sees potential in him. So he sets about enticing his pupil down the difficult road of erudition. First he must create a bond with the youth. He will gain his trust by joining the student where the student is most comfortable and unthreatened. Thus the tutor chooses an exhilarating walk in the early morning cold.

They come to a pond. The apprentice impulsively dives into its icy depths and begins swimming its length, preferring the physical challenge, one that he knows he can master and escape for a time the embarrassment of ignorance he's apt to feel with his tutor in the cognitive realm. Left on the shore, the scholar gazes at his pupil, hoping that this is the place where they shall meet, where the bond will be created. Without pondering his own physical limitations, he plunges into the rough chill of the waters and drowns.

I still see myself in that silly bathtub, the water gone cold, blubbering over the death of a fictitious teacher, and sharing with his pupil the remorse of a missed opportunity, the loss of a mentor.

Hesse's novel left me with a lasting admiration for the teacher who reaches more than halfway to capture the imagination of a novice and crosses the chasm, whether it be generational, cultural, class, or gender, to work together in shaping a discipline.

As I learn who my students are, it is each student's story that becomes the study, myself the pupil. Their uniqueness changes the nuance of the didactic, the approach to the patient. Family practice residents have contributed to the writing of this book, enriching its repertoire.

Its earliest form was a collaborative effort among doctors and nurses. Its aim was to emphasize the geriatric patient's independence and individuality. Multiple disciplines in concert with medicine are needed to achieve this, hence the "team management" sections of this book.

Dan Onion asked me to develop the next in a series of books based on the format he used in his book, *The Little Black Book of Primary Care*. Having learned a great deal from Dan's scientific approach to medicine, one which supplied references for current controversies, I could see the utility of such a geriatric manual. Dennis McCullough, a mentor since our first meeting at the Chapel Hill Family Practice Fellowship, has provided wise pearls of family practice experience. During the last legs of the book's production, I was diagnosed with breast cancer. Dennis' support and detailed review of the page proofs allowed for its timely completion.

One day this summer while sitting along side my own pond, recuperating from chemotherapy, I was visited by a resident who had come to invoke a resurgence of my bone marrow. It was her notion that an exhilarating swim would do the trick. My fears of deep water made me an unwilling student and encumbered her cure. Eventually, she coached me across the pond and back, keeping me afloat as my colleagues have done these past months.

I hope you, the reader, whether primary care provider, student, or resident, will find what we've put together useful, knowing all along that your patients will be most helped by what you bring of yourself to the patient encounter.

K. G.

ADDENDUM

My friend, colleague, and coauthor could not have fully realized how I have always relished the extra innings of the game, the tie-breaker, the overtime period. When I was asked to enter this process, I was awed by the quality and tone of Dr. Gershman's text, accomplished over months and months of hard labor—the first seven innings. Helping to bring

Karen's work to print has been a thrill and a pleasure. I have enjoyed the opportunity to draw on my love of working with older folks and their families and with our health care team at Kendal at Hanover, a continuing care retirement community near the Dartmouth-Hitchcock Medical Center.

The perspectives that I have gained from trying to be a team player in geriatrics have substantially complemented my understanding of "diseases" in elderly people. Many answers to clinical situations are to be found in interdisciplinary discussions and in time-requiring "processing" with patients and their families—this book of information is only the starting point for this clinical work. I encourage the reader to listen, discuss, and work slowly over time in these wonderful and complicated partnerships in order to bring the very best care and caring to patients.

D. M.

Acknowledgments

Several primary care providers have contributed to the writing of various sections of this book. They include:

Diana Berger, MD, Hanover, NH	Gout
Sandy Colt, GNP, Maine Veterans' Home	UTIs/Constipation
Steve Diaz, MD, MaineGeneral Medical Center	External Feeding
Rich Entel, MD, MDFPR*	AIDS
Lance Feray, DO, MDFPR	Arthritis
Rod Forrey, PA, MDFPR	Anxiety; Neuroleptic Malignant Syndrome
Kathryn Galbraith, MD, MDFPR	Osteoporosis
Chris Lutrzykowski, MD, MDFPR	AIDS
James MacDonald, MD, MDFPR	ETOH Abuse
Catherine Neilsen, MD, MDFPR	Pneumonia; Influenza; Elderly Abuse
Daniel K. Onion, MD, MDFPR	Cardiology
Michelle Rebelsky, MD, MDFPR	Ethics
James A. Schneid, MD, MDFPR	Diabetes Mellitus

Special thanks to Marsha Fretwell, MD for reviewing the manuscript and to Julie Roullard and Nancy Greenier for their library expertise. I would also like to thank Davene Fitch, Diane Hall, and Sharon Peacock for their help in the preparation for the book.

*Maine-Dartmouth Family Practice Residency.

Medical Abbreviations

AA	Alcoholics Anonymous	BP	Blood pressure
AADLs	Advanced activities of daily living	BPH	Benign prostatic hypertrophy
ABG	Arterial blood gases	BSOO	Bilateral salpingo-oophorectomy
ABW	Actual body weight		
ac	Before meals	BUN	Blood urea nitrogen
ACE	Angiotensin-converting enzyme	bx	Biopsy
ACTH	Adrenocorticotropic hormone	CABG	Coronary artery bypass graft
ADLs	Activities of daily living	CAD	Coronary artery disease
AFB	Acid-fast bacilli	cal	Calories
Afib	Atrial fibrillation	CBC	Complete blood cell count
Aflut	Atrial flutter	CEA	Carcinoembryonic antigen
ALT	SGPT; alanine aminotransferase	chem	Chemistries
		chemo rx	Chemotherapy
ANA	Antinuclear antibody	CHF	Congestive heart failure
AP	Anterior-posterior	CML	Chronic myelocytic leukemia
ARDS	Adult respiratory distress syndrome		
		CN	Cranial nerve
As	Arsenic	CNS	Central nervous system
AS	Aortic stenosis	Complc	Complications
ASA	Aspirin	COPD	Chronic obstructive lung disease
ASCVD	Arteriosclerotic cardiovascular disease		
		CPAP	Continuous positive airway pressure
ASHD	Arteriosclerotic heart disease		
		CPK	Creatine phosphokinase
AST	SGOT; aspartate aminotransferase	CPR	Cardiopulmonary resuscitation
asx	Asymptomatic	Cr	Creatinine
AV	Arteriovenous; or atrioventricular	CRP	C-reactive protein
		crs	Course
avg	Average	CSF	Cerebrospinal fluid
		CT	Computed tomography
		CVA	Cerebrovascular accident
bcp's	Birth control pills	CVP	Central venous pressure
BE	Barium enema		
bid	Twice a day	d	Day
bm	Bowel movement	dB	Decibel

DI	Diabetes insipidus	gtts	Drops
DM	Diabetes mellitus	gu	Genitourinary
D$_5$S	Dextrose 5% in saline		
DSM	Diagnostic and statistical manual	h	Hour
		HCl	Hydrochloride
DTRs	Deep tendon reflexes	hct	Hematocrit
DVT	Deep vein thrombosis	HDL	High-density lipoprotein
dx	Diagnosis or diagnostic	Hg	Mercury
		hgb	Hemoglobin
ECT	Electroconvulsive therapy	HgbA$_{1C}$	Hemoglobin A$_{1C}$ level
EDTA	Ethylenediaminetetra-acetate	5HIAA	5-Hydroxyindoleacetic acid
		HIV	Human immunodeficiency virus
EEG	Electroencephalogram		
EF	Ejection fraction	HMG-CoA	Hepatic hydroxymethyl-glutaryl–coenzyme A
EKG	Electrocardiogram		
Epidem	Epidemiology	h/o	History of
ER	Estrogen receptors; or emergency room	hs	At bedtime
		HT	Hypertension
ERCP	Endoscopic retrograde cho-langiopancreatography	hx	History
		Hz	Hertz
ERT	Estrogen replacement therapy	IADLs	Instrumental or intermedi-ate activities of daily living
ESR	Erythrocyte sedimentation rate		
ETOH	Ethanol	IBW	Ideal body weight
ETT	Exercise tolerance test	ICU	Intensive care unit
		IHSS	Idiopathic hypertrophic subaortic stenosis
F	Female, or Fahrenheit	IL	Interleukin
FBS	Fasting blood sugar	im	Intramuscular
Fe	Iron	INH	Isoniazid
FEV$_1$	Forced expiratory vital capacity in 1 second	INR	International normalized ratio
FSH	Follicle-stimulating hor-mone	IPG	Impedance plethysmog-raphy
f/u	Follow-up	iv	Intravenous
FVC	Forced vital capacity	IVP	Intravenous pyelography
GABA	γ-Aminobutyric acid	JVD	Jugular venous distension
GE	Gastroesophageal		
GFR	Glomerular filtration rate	L	Liter; or left
gi	Gastrointestinal	Lab	Laboratory tests
gm	Gram	LBBB	Left bundle branch block

LDH	Lactate dehydrogenase	NNT	Number needed to treat
LDL	Low-density lipoprotein	NPH	Normal-pressure hydro-cephalus
LFTs	Liver function tests		
LH	Luteinizing hormone	NSAID	Nonsteroidal anti-inflam-matory drug
LP	Lumbar puncture		
LS	Lumbosacral	NSR	Normal sinus rhythm
LV	Left ventricle		
LVH	Left ventricular hyper-trophy	OGTT	Oral glucose tolerance test
lytes	Electrolytes	OTC	Over the counter
m	Meter		
M	Male	PA	Pernicious anemia; or pul-monary artery
MAO	Monoamine oxidase		
MCV	Mean corpuscular volume	PAP	Pulmonary artery pressure
meds	Medications	PAT	Paroxysmal atrial tachy-cardia
METS	Metabolic equivalents		
Mg	Magnesium	Pathophys	Pathophysiology
MI	Myocardial infarction; or mitral insufficiency	Pb	Lead
		PCP	*Pneumocystis carinii* pneu-monia
min	Minute		
mL	Milliliter	PCWP	Pulmonary capillary wedge pressure
mmHg	Millimeters of mercury		
MMSE	Mini-Mental State Exam	PE	Pulmonary embolism
mo	Month	PET	Positron emission tomog-raphy
MOM	Milk of magnesia		
MR	Mitral regurgitation	PFTs	Pulmonary function tests
MRA	Magnetic resonance angiog-raphy		
		PMNLs	Polymorphonuclear leuko-cytes
MRI	Magnetic resonance imaging		
MS	Multiple sclerosis; or mitral stenosis	PMR	Polymyalgia rheumatica
		ppd	Packs per day
Musc-skel	Musculoskeletal	PPD	Tuberculin skin test; puri-fied protein derivative
μgm	Microgram		
		po	By mouth
		pos	Positive
Na	Sodium	postop	Postoperative
NA	Narcotics Anonymous	pr	By rectum
neg	Negative	pRBBB	Partial right bundle branch block
NG	Nasogastric		
NH	Nursing home	preop	Preoperative
NIDDM	Non-insulin-dependent dia-betes mellitus	PSA	Prostate-specific antigen
		PT	Prothrombin time
nl	Normal	pt(s)	Patient(s)

Medical Abbreviations **xi**

PTH	Parathyroid hormone	SR	Slow release
PTT	Partial thromboplastin time	SSRI	Selective serotonin reuptake inhibitor
PUD	Peptic ulcer disease	SSS	Sick sinus syndrome
PUVA	Psoralen + UVA light	SVR	Systemic vascular resistance
PVC	Premature ventricular tachycardia	SVT	Supraventricular tachycardia
PVR	Postvoid residual	sx	Symptoms
q	Every		
qd	Every day	T°	Fever/temperature
qid	4 times a day	T_3	Triiodothyronine
qod	Every other day	T_4	Thyroxine
quad	Quadricep	tab	Tablet
		TAH	Total abdominal hysterectomy
R	Right; or respirations		
RA	Rheumatoid arthritis	TB	Tuberculosis
RBBB	Right bundle branch block	TENS	Transcutaneous electrical stimulation
rbc	Red blood cell		
rehab	Rehabilitation	TIA	Transient ischemic attack
REM	Rapid eye movement	TIBC	Total iron binding capacity
r/o	Rule out	Tm/S	Trimethoprim/sulfa
RV	Right ventricle	TNG	Nitroglycerin
rx	Treatment	TPA	Tissue plasminogen activator
sc	Subcutaneous	TPN	Total parenteral nutrition
sec	Seconds	TSH	Thyroid-stimulating hormone
sens	Sensitivity		
si	Signs	tsp	Teaspoon
SIADH	Syndrome of inappropriate antidiuretic hormone		
		UA	Urinalysis
sl	Sublingual	UBW	Usual body weight
SLE	Systemic lupus erythematosus	UGI	Upper gastrointestinal
		UPEP	Urine protein electrophoresis
soln	Solution		
s/p	Status post	URI	Upper respiratory infection
specif	Specificity		
SPECT	Single-photon emission computed tomography	US	Ultrasound
		UTI	Urinary tract infection
		UV	Ultraviolet
SPEP	Serum protein electrophoresis	UVA	Ultraviolet A
		UVB	Ultraviolet B

VDRL	Serologic test for syphilis (Venereal Disease Research Lab)	w	With
		w/o	Without
		w/u	Workup
vit	Vitamin	wbc	White blood cell
vs	Versus	wk	Week
Vtach	Ventricular tachycardia	WPW	Wolff-Parkinson-White syndrome
		yr	Year

Journals and Other Reference Abbreviations

(Journal abbreviation is followed by year, volume, and page or issue number)

ACP J Club	American College of Physicians Journal Club
Acta Neurol Scand	Acta Neurologica Scandinavica
Acta Psychiatr Scand	Acta Psychiatrica Scandinavica
Adv Wound Care	Advances in Wound Healing
Age Aging	Age and Aging
Alzheimer Dis Assoc Disord	Alzheimer Disease and Associated Disorders
Am Fam Phys	American Family Physician
Am Heart J	American Heart Journal
Am J Cardiol	American Journal of Cardiology
Am J Clin Oncol	American Journal of Clinical Oncology
Am J Gastroenterol	American Journal of Gastroenterology
Am J Ger Psychiatry	American Journal of Geriatric Psychiatry
Am J Hlth Syst Pharmacol	American Journal of Health-System Pharmacy
Am J Hosp Pharm	American Journal of Hospital Pharmacy
Am J Hypertens	American Journal of Hypertension
Am J Kidney Dis	American Journal of Kidney Disease
Am J Med	American Journal of Medicine
Am J Nurs	American Journal of Nursing
Am J Obgyn	American Journal of Obstetrics and Gynecology
Am J Phys Med Rehab	American Journal of Physical Medicine and Rehabilitation
Am J Psychiatry	American Journal of Psychiatry
Am J Pub Hlth	American Journal of Public Health
Am Rev Respir Dis	American Review of Respiratory Diseases

Ann EM	Annals of Emergency Medicine
Ann IM	Annals of Internal Medicine
Ann Neurol	Annals of Neurology
Ann Oncol	Annals of Oncology
Ann Pharmacother	Annals of Pharmacotherapy
Ann Rev Pub Hlth	Annual Review of Public Health
Ann Thorac Surg	Annals of Thoracic Surgery
Arch Fam Med	Archives of Family Medicine
Arch IM	Archives of Internal Medicine
Arch Ophthalm	Archives of Ophthalmology
Arch Phys Med Rehab	Archives of Physical Medicine and Rehabilitation
Arch Sex Behav	Archives of Sexual Behavior
Arch Surg	Archives of Surgery
Arth Rheum	Arthritis and Rheumatism
Aust NZ J Surg	Australia and New Zealand Journal of Surgery
Basic Res Cardiol	Basic Research in Cardiology
Biol Psychiatry	Biological Psychiatry
BMJ	British Medical Journal
Bone Marrow Transplant	Bone Marrow Transplantation
Bone Miner	Bone and Mineral
Br J Cancer	British Journal of Cancer
Br J Psychiatry	British Journal of Psychiatry
Br J Surg	British Journal of Surgery
Bull Rheum Dis	Bulletin on the Rheumatic Diseases
CA	CA: A Cancer Journal for Clinicians
Can J Psychiatry	Canadian Journal of Psychiatry
Cancer Causes Control	Cancer Causes and Control
Cancer Nurs	Cancer Nursing
Cancer Pract	Cancer Practice
Circ	Circulation
Clin Diabetes	Clinical Diabetes
Clin Endocrinol	Clinical Endocrinology (Oxford)
Clin Ger Med	Clinics in Geriatric Medicine
Clin Gerontol	Clinical Gerontology
Clin Orthop	Clinical Orthopedics and Related Research

Clin Pharmacol Ther	Clinical Pharmacology and Therapeutics
Clin Symp	Clinical Symposia
Consult Pharm	Consultant Pharmacist
Convuls Ther	Convulsive Therapy
Curr Concepts Cerebro Dis	Current Concepts of Cerebrovascular Disease
Curr Opin Neurol	Current Opinion in Neurology
Curr Probl Cancer	Current Problems in Cancer
Curr Probl Cardiol	Current Problems in Cardiology
Diabetes Metab Rev	Diabetes/Metabolism Reviews
Dis Mo	Disease-a-Month
Ear Hear	Ear and Hearing
Emerg Med Clin N Am	Emergency Medicine Clinics of North America
Endocr Rev	Endocrine Reviews
Eur J Cancer	European Journal of Cancer
Eur J Surg Oncol	European Journal of Surgical Oncology
Eur Respir J	European Respiratory Journal
Exp Aging Res	Experimental Aging Research
Fortschr Neurol Psychiatrie	Fortschritte der Neurologie-Psychiatrie
Gastroenterol Int	Gastroenterology International
Gastrointest Endosc Clin N Am	Gastrointestinal Endoscopy Clinics of North America
Ger Clin N Am	Geriatric Clinics of North America
Ger Med Today	Geriatric Medicine Today
Ger Rev Syllabus	Geriatric Review Syllabus
Gerontol	Gerontologist
Gerontol Clin	Gerontologia Clinica
Heart Lung	Heart and Lung
Hlth Serv Res	Health Services Research
Horm Metab Res	Hormone and Metabolic Research
Hosp Pract	Hospital Practice
Inf Contr Hosp Epidem	Infection Control and Hospital Epidemiology

Int J Aging Hum Dev	International Journal of Aging and Human Development
Int J Psychiatr Med	International Journal of Psychiatry in Medicine
J Acoustic Soc Am	Journal of the Acoustical Society of America
J Acquir Immun Defic Syndr	Journal of the Acquired Immune Deficiency Syndromes and Human Retrovirology
Jama	Journal of the American Medical Association
J Am Board Fam Pract	Journal of the American Board of Family Practice
J Am Coll Cardiol	Journal of the American College of Cardiology
J Am Diet Assoc	Journal of the American Dietetic Association
J Am Ger Soc	Journal of the American Geriatrics Society
J Am Optom Assoc	Journal of the American Optometric Association
J Bone Joint Surg Am	Journal of Bone and Joint Surgery (American vol)
J Chronic Dis	Journal of Chronic Diseases
J Clin Invest	Journal of Clinical Investigation
J Clin Oncol	Journal of Clinical Oncology
J Clin Psychiatry	Journal of Clinical Psychiatry
J Clin Psychopharmacol	Journal of Clinical Psychopharmacology
J Comm Health	Journal of Community Health
J Emerg Med	Journal of Emergency Medicine
J Endocrinol Metab	Journal of Endocrinology and Metabolism
J Endourol	Journal of Endourology
J Fam Pract	Journal of Family Practice
J Gen IM	Journal of General Internal Medicine
J Ger Psychiatry	Journal of Geriatric Psychiatry
J Ger Psychiatry Neurol	Journal of Geriatric Psychiatry and Neurology

J Gerontol	Journal of Gerontology
J Gerontol Med Sci	Journals of Gerontology Series A Biological Sciences and Medical Sciences
J Gerontol Nurs	Journal of Gerontological Nursing
J Hypertens	Journal of Hypertension
J Hypertens Suppl	Journal of Hypertension Supplement
J Intern Med	Journal of Internal Medicine
J Natl Cancer Inst	Journal of the National Cancer Institute
J Neurol Sci	Journal of the Neurological Sciences
J Neurosurg	Journal of Neurosurgery
J Optom Assoc	Journal of the American Optometric Association
J Psycho Nurs	Journal of Psychological Nursing
J Rheum	Journal of Rheumatology
J Trauma	Journal of Trauma
J Urol	Journal of Urology
Leuk Lymphoma	Leukemia and Lymphoma
Life Sci	Life Sciences
Mayo Clin Proc	Mayo Clinic Proceedings
Md State Med Assoc J	Maryland State Medical Association Journal
Med Aud Dig	Medical Audio Digest
Med Clin N Am	Medical Clinics of North America
Med Let Drugs Ther	Medical Letter on Drugs and Therapeutics
Milbank Q	Milbank Quarterly
Mmwr	Morbidity and Mortality Weekly Report
Mod Concepts Cardiovasc Dis	Modern Concepts of Cardiovascular Disease
Natl Ctr Hlth Stat	National Center for Health Statistics
Nejm	New England Journal of Medicine
Neurol	Neurology
Nurs Home Med	Nursing Home Medicine
Nurs Home Pract	Nursing Home Practice

Nutr Rev	Nutrition Reviews
Obgyn	Obstetrics and Gynecology
Ophthalm	Ophthalmology
Osteoporos Int	Osteoporosis International
Ped Derm	Pediatric Dermatology
Phys Postgrad Med	Physicians Postgraduate Medicine
Prim Care	Primary Care
Prog Clin Biol Res	Progress in Clinical and Biological Research
Psych Ann	Psychiatric Annals
Psychiatr Clin N Am	Psychiatric Clinics of North America
Psychol Med	Psychological Medicine
Psychosom	Psychosomatics
Radiol Clin N Am	Radiologic Clinics of North America
Sci Am	Scientific American
Sci Am Med	Scientific American Medicine
Semin Oncol	Seminars in Oncology
Semin Spine Surg	Seminars in Spine Surgery
South Med J	Southern Medical Journal
Surg Clin N Am	Surgical Clinics of North America
Surv Ophthalmol	Survey of Ophthalmology
Urol Clin N Am	Urologic Clinics of North America

Notice

We have made every attempt to summarize accurately and concisely a multitude of references. However, the reader is reminded that times and medical knowledge change, transcription or understanding error is always possible, and crucial details are omitted whenever such a comprehensive distillation as this is attempted in limited space. The primary purpose of this compilation is to cite literature on various sides of controversial issues; knowing where "truth" lies is usually difficult. The book is not intended to be comprehensive, as the preface explains. We cannot, therefore, guarantee that every bit of information is absolutely accurate or complete. The reader should affirm that cited recommendations are reasonable still by reading the original articles and checking other sources including local consultants as well as recent literature before applying them.

1. Common Geriatric Problems

DYSFUNCTION IN ELDERLY

Cause: Loss of physical, mental, social function, excessive family burden (Gerontol 1980;20:649)

Epidem: In 1985, 20% of elderly were disabled; by 2060, 30% will be disabled (J Gerontol 1992;47.S253); among individuals 65 yr and older, >20% have difficulty walking a half mile, >30% have difficulty doing heavy housework, 50% have difficulty pulling or pushing large objects such as furniture; 30% community elders live alone: M/F ratio = 1:3; the remainder live in family settings: 54% w spouse, 13% w children, 3% w nonrelatives (DHHS Publc 1990; PF3029912900 d996)

  50% of all long-term care payments come from individual and family finances, most of which are spent on NH care; Medicaid coverage during the first year of NH placement = 20% but overall >90% of all public funds for NH care provided by Medicaid; Medicare pays for skilled home-care services, but only 3% of NH care; private long-term care insurance pays 2% of NH care (Gerontol 1990;30:7,21)

Sx: Loss of self-care/independent living skills

Si: Inability to read 20/40; inability to answer short, whispered question such as "What is your name?"; urinary incontinence; weight below acceptable range for height; inability to recall 3 objects after 1 min; often sad or depressed; can't get out of bed, make own meals, do own shopping; trouble with stairs, bathtubs, rugs, lighting; doesn't know where to call in emergency or if ill (Ann IM 1990;112:699); inability to touch back of head with both hands, touch back of waist, or contralateral hip; inability to sit and touch toe of shoe; no grip strength (J Fam Pract 1993;17:429)

ADLs: Katz functional assessment (Gerontol 1970;10:20) records loss of independence in 6 skills (in the order in which they are lost: bathing, dressing, toileting, transferring, continence, feeding); usually they are regained in the reverse order; assess actual capacity, not reported performance (Nejm 1990;322:1207); Mahoney and Barthel ADL scale has more specific questions (Md State Med Assoc J 1965;14:61); speed and pain in performing ADLs in arthritis pts (J Chronic Dis 1978;31:557); use of rehabilitation for ADLs (Arch Phys Med Rehab 1988;69:337)

Instrumental activities of daily living (IADLs), more complex activities like shopping, seeking transportation, preparing food, climbing stairs, and managing finances, housework, telephone, meds, and job (Fillenbaum IADLs–J Am Ger Soc 1985;33:698); mnemonic: SHAFT: shopping, housework, accounting, food preparation, transportation (Mayo Clin Proc 1995;70:891)

Other IADL scales: home assessment (Clin Ger Med 1991;7:677); nutrition (Am Fam Phys 1993;48:1395); driving (Clin Ger Med 1993;9:349), states where standard vision tests required for driver license renewal have fewer fatalities, whereas states requiring cognitive function test show no difference in fatalities (Jama 1995; 274:1026); identify older pts at risk for functional decline after acute medical illness and hospitalization w scoring system based on Mini Mental State Exam (MMSE), IADLs, and age (J Am Ger Soc 1996;44:251); advanced ADLs (AADLs) in community-dwelling elderly

Crs: For every 5 adults with 5–6 limitations in ADLs, 1 pt may be expected to improve in all ADLs in 2 yr (Milbank Q 1990;68:445); pts who have trouble performing IADLs have 12× the baseline probability of developing dementia (J Am Ger Soc 1992;40:1129)

Cmplc: NH placement; Medicaid eligibility for NH admission requires a medical or behavioral dx, plus 2 impaired ADLs; caregiver burnout: 70% of primary caregivers are middle-aged, married women, 30% are elderly themselves (Gerontol 1987;27:616); prevalence of depression among caregivers is 30%–50% (J Gerontol 1990; 45:P181)

Lab: CBC, TSH, routine blood chemistries

Rx:

Team Management: Rehab; change medical regimen so as not to inhibit function; solicit community services; be vigilant about underlying depression

FALLS IN THE ELDERLY

Ann IM 1994;121:442; Nejm 1994;331:821; J Am Ger Soc 1995;43: 1146; Nejm 1990;322:1441; Rubenstein LZ, UCLA intensive geriatric review course, 1996

Cause:

Intrinsic:

- Visual: cataracts, acuity loss, glare, dark adaptation (J Am Ger Soc 1991;39:1194; Nejm 1991;324:1326)
- Vestibular: previous ear infection, ear surgery, aminoglycosides, quinidine, furosemide (Lasix)
- Proprioceptive: peripheral neuropathy, cervical degeneration; one-third of elderly have abnormal position sense (Jama 1988; 259:1190)
- CNS: stroke, Parkinson's, NPH
- Cognitive: dementia
- Musc-skel: deconditioning, lower extremity weakness, eg, severe arthritis (Nejm 1988;319:1701); leg weakness imparts 5× the risk of fall compared with balance or gait problem, which imparts only 3× the risk of fall; knee extension (quads) and ankle plantar flexion (gastrocnemius and soleus) strength contribute to gait velocity and step length; foot problems like thick nails, calluses, bunions, toe deformities, ill-fitting shoes (J Am Ger Soc 1988;36:266)
- Drugs (>4 meds a risk factor) especially long-acting benzodiazepines, tricyclics, and phenothiazines (Nejm 1987;316:363)

NH falls (Ann IM 1994;121:442): 20% are cardiovascular, eg, hypotension—drug-induced, postprandial, postural, bradycardia (J Gerontol 1991;46:M114); 5% due to acute illness like pneumonia, febrile illness, UTI, CHF (Am J Med 1986;80:429); only 3% falls from overwhelming intrinsic event, eg, syncope, seizure, stroke, psychoactive drugs (Nejm 1992;327:168)

Extrinsic: Majority occur with mild-moderate activity, eg, walking, stepping up, stepping down, changing position; 70% at home,10% on stairs (descending > ascending) (Age Aging 1979; 8:251); >50% due to environmental hazards, eg, cords, furniture, small objects, optical patterns on escalators, stairs, floors (Clin Ger Med 1985;1:555)

NH: (Paradoxically) restraints (Ann IM 1992;116:369); higher fall rate during shift changes and when staffing ratios inadequate (J Am Ger Soc 1987;35:503)

Epidem: Accidents 5th leading cause of death in elderly; falls constitute two-thirds of accidental deaths; two-thirds of falls are preventable; 33% of elderly (>65) living in the *community* fall each year; females > males, whites > blacks (Nejm 1994;330:1555); active elderly at greater risk than frail elderly for injury (J Am Ger Soc 1991;39:46)

Over 50% of all *NH* pts fall during their stay because of greater frailty but rate may be high because better reporting (J Am Ger Soc 1988;36:266)

Pathophys: Fracture risk from falls increased in elderly because of decreased energy absorption capability of tissue and impaired protective responses like reaction time, muscle strength, level of alertness, cognition (J Gerontol 1991;46:M164)

Falls from standing height provide sufficient energy to fracture hip (Nejm 1991;332:1326; Jama 1994;271:128); more likely to fracture a wrist than a hip when falling forward bracing a fall; falling backward more hazardous because of risk of breaking hip (J Am Ger Soc 1993;41:1226)

In old age the strategy for maintaining balance after a slip changes from weight shifting at hip when younger to rapid forward stepping when older (Rubenstein LZ, 1996)

Sx: H/o hypotensive sx posturally, postprandially, on micturition; may have h/o PAT, SSS, AS, hemiplegia, neuropathy, seizures, anemia, hypothyroidism, poor nutritional status, ETOH abuse, intercurrent illness (UTI, pneumonia, CHF); or use of antihypertensives, antidepressants, sedatives, hypoglycemics, phenothiazines, or carbamazepine

Si: Evaluate environment: stairs, floors (slippery from urine, high-polish linoleum, thick-pile rugs), low-lying furniture, pets, shower, lighting, stairway handrails, toilet grab bars, footwear, slippers

Tinetti Gait/Balance Assessment:

Balance:

- Upon immediate standing (if abnormal, consider myopathy, arthritis, Parkinson's, postural hypotension, deconditioning, hip disease, hemiparesis)
- With eyes closed and feet together (if abnormal, consider multisensory deficit or diminished proprioception)
- If unstable with sternal nudge, turning 360 degrees (consider Par-

kinson's, NPH, CNS disease, back problems, cervical spondylosis); especially important to determine prior to beginning exercise classes

- As sitting down (if abnormal, consider impaired vision, proximal myopathy, ataxia)
- When turning neck (if abnormal, consider cervical arthritis or spondylosis, vertebrobasilar insufficiency)
- When reaching up, bending down, standing on one leg, screening test for higher-functioning individuals in the community; if unable to perform, at risk for falls at home (J Am Ger Soc 1986;34:119)

Gait (Table 1-1): 6% of F >65, 38% >85; 63% NH residents have gait abnormality (J Am Ger Soc 1996;44:434); timed 8-foot walk and other lower extremity function tests predict mobility-related ADL disability in 4 yr (Nejm 1995;332:556); NH pt's self-selected gait speed and perception of physical disability and predictive of functional loss (J Am Ger Soc 1995;43:93); comfortable walking speed better predictor than treadmill test of cardiac status in pts w CHF; changes w normal aging: broader-based, smaller steps, diminished arm swing, stooped posture, slower turning

- Step height: Frontal lobe gait, seen in vascular dementia, most common gait abnormality: wide-based, slightly flexed, small shuffling steps, hesitant steps, can't initiate step, "glued to floor" (Nejm 1990;322:1441)

  Spastic gait, seen in stroke w circumduction, scrape foot along floor, hand-arm spasticity; also seen w cervical stenosis and myopathy w bilateral circumduction, sometimes increased urinary frequency and urgency (J Am Ger Soc 1996;44:A)

  Parkinsonian gait, lacks arm swing, turns en bloc (moves whole body when turns), hesitation, gets stuck while walking ("freezing"), especially in open spaces like doorways, festination (involuntary increase in speed of walking in attempt to catch up with displaced center of gravity forward), 4th most common gait abnormality

  NPH, short steps, decreased velocity of stride length and associated shoulder movements, increased sway, poor balance, difficulty turning; overlap between NPH and vascular etiologies, eg, hydrocephalus from stroke may account for similar gait abnormalities (J Am Ger Soc 1996;44:434)

  Steppage gait w foot slap seen in distal motor neuropathies

Table 1-1. Tinetti Gait Assessment

Gait Abnormality	Type of Gait	Description	Etiology	Dx/Rx
Step height/length	Spastic	Wide-based, slightly flexed, small shuffling steps, hesitant steps, can't initiate step, "glued to floor"	Vascular dementia	Trochanteric pads decrease hip fx
		Circumduction, scrape foot along floor, hand-arm spasticity	Stroke	Surgery
		Bilateral circumduction, sometimes increase urinary frequency and urgency	Spinal stenosis	Surgery
	NPH	Short steps, decreased velocity of stride length and associated shoulder movements, increased sway, poor balance, difficulty turning		Shunt
	Parkinson's	Lacks arm swing, turn en bloc (moves whole body when turns), hesitation, gets stuck while walking especially in open spaces like doorways, festination		Front-wheeled walker
	Steppage	W foot slap	Seen in distal motor neuropathies	Foot orthotics

		Description	Associated with	Findings/Treatment
Path deviation	Vestibular	Broad-based foot stamping, pt looks at feet Unsteady on one side and then the other	Sensory ataxia Peripheral neuropathy	Pos Rhomberg/↓ position/vibration sensitivity at ankle
	Weakness	Slow unsteady swagger, use furniture to grab onto when walking	Deconditioning	Atrophy, 2/5 strength
Postural sway	Cerebellar	Wide-based, irregular, unsteady, veering, truncal titubation	MS	
	Waddling	Broad based	Seen with severe arthritis, myositis, PMR	
	Antalgic	Seen with arthritis of hip when cane held incorrectly on same side Throwing trunk out over affected hip, resulting in stress on hip and low back		Analgesics, hip replacement
Hysterical		Hemiparesis without circumduction, hemiparetic arm normal during walking, good strength lying down but ataxia when walking, staggering a long time to get to opposite wall, tightrope walking, pt drags person assisting them down to the ground		Reassurance

- Path deviation: observe from behind, one foot at a time in relation to midline; abnormal path deviation in:

  Vestibular gait, seen with sensory ataxia, 2nd most common gait abnormality, broad-based, foot stamping, pt looks at feet; and peripheral neuropathy gait, 3rd most common, unsteady on one side and then the other, pos Romberg (pt unable to maintain balance w eyes closed)

  Muscle weakness, slow unsteady swagger, uses furniture to grab onto when walking

- Postural sway: observe from behind for truncal side-to-side motion; w:

  Cerebellar gait, 5th most common gait disturbance, wide-based, irregular, unsteady, veering, truncal titubation (shimmying of thorax with respect to the rest of the body)

  Antalgic gait, seen with arthritis of hip when cane held incorrectly on same side, throwing trunk out over affected hip resulting in stress on hip and low back (Ger Med Today 1985;4:47; J Am Ger Soc 1996;44:434)

  Waddling gait, broad-based, seen with severe arthritis, myositis, PMR

- Hysterical gait: hemiparesis without circumduction, hemiparetic arm normal during walking, good strength lying down but ataxia when walking, staggering a long time to get to opposite wall, gait resembles attempts at tightrope walking, pt drags person assisting them down to the ground, not known to occur in pts >70 yr (J Am Ger Soc 1996;44:434)

Cmplc: Clustering of falls associated with high 6-mo mortality (Age Aging 1977;6:201), 6% fracture some bone, one-fourth being hip fractures (J Am Ger Soc 1995;43:1146); 2% of injurious falls are fatal, of those 13% die from pulmonary embolus; white men 85 yr and older have highest rate of deaths attributable to falls, exceeding 180/100 000 population (Ann Rev Pub Hlth 1992;13: 489); 5% serious soft tissue injury (Nejm 1988;319:1701)

Prolonged lies while waiting for help (<10% of falls), if >1 h may cause dehydration, pressure sores, rhabdomyolysis, pneumonia (Jama 1993;268:65)

25% of fallers subsequently avoid ADLs, IADLs, and AADLs for fear of falling again (J Gerontol 1994;49:M140; Nejm 1988;319:1701)

NH admissions (Am J Pub Hlth 1992;82:395): Increased use of health care services (Med Care 1992;30:587); ~50% pts that are hospitalized for falls may end up in NHs (Emerg Med Clin N Am 1990;8:309)

Lab: Routine w/u: CBC w differential, UA, chem screen, stool guaiacs, TSH, vit B_{12}, and ESR (r/o PMR), EKG, chest xray, and/or CT as hx indicates

Noninvasive: No need to Holter monitor; prevalence of ventricular arrhythmia is 82% in both fallers and nonfallers; no sx reported with these arrhythmias (J Am Ger Soc 1989;37:430)

Rx:

Prevention: (Programs reduce falls by one-third–Nejm 1994;331: 821)

- Assessing falls in elderly (J Am Ger Soc 1993;41:309,315,479); Medicare allowable charges for the evaluation of falls: CBC, EKG, MRI, neurologic, orthopedic, physical therapy consultation, safety and functional evaluation of pt's home (Jama 1996; 276:59); w questionnaire assess those at risk of immobility because of fear of falling (J Gerontol Med Sci 1995;45:P239)
- Minimizing number of meds using lowest possible doses
- Treating osteoporosis with estrogen replacement (Nejm 1993; 329:1141; Am J Med 1993:95:75S)
- Exercise programs (Nejm 1994;330:1769) to increase muscle strength and flexibility (FICSIT trials Jama 1995;273:1341; J Am Ger Soc 1996;44:513)

  Resistance training to improve weakness, which may be more of a limiting factor than endurance (J Am Ger Soc 1994;42:937)

  Flexibility programs to increase range of motion for tight hip flexors common in thoracic kyphosis, tightness in hip abductors and adductors

  Balance and gait training, especially getting in and out of chairs, turning around; NH standard physical therapy is of moderate benefit (Jama 1994;271:519); perturbation training (pushes in different directions to stimulate postural responses) more useful in community setting

  Endurance training to help compensate for extra energy cost gait dysfunctions impose; using crutches requires 60% more energy than normal walking; 3-wk bed rest decreases VO_2 max by 27%

- Tai Chi: cardiorespiratory function better among older Tai Chi practitioners (J Am Ger Soc 1995;43:1222); Tai Chi decreases falls (J Am Ger Soc 1996;44:489,498)

- Assistive aids: 23% of noninstitutionalized elderly use assistive aids; of those who use assistive aids, 49% use a cane (70% use incorrectly), 24% use a walker, 12% use a wheelchair (Natl Ctr Hlth Stat 1992;217:1)

  Walker use s/p hip fracture (advance 20–30 cm, then move weak leg first)

  Front-wheeled walker for Parkinson's avoids retropulsion and tripping

  Cane use s/p hip fracture only if ipsilateral upper extremity and contralateral lower extremity are strong; <25% of pt's weight should be placed on cane; when going up or down stairs, keep good leg up higher, ie, "up with good, down with bad"; although ipsilateral cane use can reduce the force acting on the hip, placing the cane in the contralateral hand is useful in relieving hip pain, watch for development of new shoulder problem with added stress (J Am Ger Soc 1996;44:434); cane height should allow 30 degrees of flexion at the pt's elbow w top of cane parallel to greater trochanter

  Trochanteric pads decrease hip fractures (Jama 1994;271:128), facilitate compliance w graduated implementation; pts are more likely to wear them if the trochanteric pads are only worn at pt-specified limited time periods (J Am Ger Soc 1993: 41:338)

- Neck collars for vertebral insufficiency (Rubenstein LZ, 1996)
- Proper shoes, high-heel shoes decrease balance in elderly women (J Am Ger Soc 1996;44:434)
- Chairs, toilet seats should have arm rests and increased seat height
- Obstacle-free, glare-free, adequately lit environment
- Avoid physical and pharmacologic restraints (Jama 1991;265: 468; Ann IM 1992;116:369); alternatives: special areas for walking, lower beds, floor pads, alarm systems (Am Fam Phys 1992; 45:763), surveillance by staff, tape player w headphones w tapes of favorite music, talking books, and family messages (Neufeld R, Phoenix, AZ, 1997); hospital alternatives: use of family visitors, professional sitters, lower beds, "functional" ICUs

GERIATRIC PHARMACOLOGY

Family practice review course, Seattle, WA, 3/95; Mayo Clin Proc 1995; 70:685

Overused Chronically Administered Drugs in *NH:* TNG patches and paste, isosorbide dinitrate; sleeping meds, antipsychotics for dementia, antidepressants; digoxin, diuretics, antihypertensives; antiepileptics; laxatives and vitamins; NSAIDs; H_2 blockers and sucralfate (Nurs Home Med 1995;3:254); 10% of all elderly hospitalizations are due to adverse drug reactions (Ann IM 1992;117: 634); most common drug-drug interactions causing side effects leading to hospitalization are diuretics, benzodiazepines, ACE inhibitors (J Am Ger Soc 1996;44:944; Ann IM 1995;123:195)

Pharmacokinetics:

Absorption: Absorption of ciprofloxacin eliminated by concomitant administration of antacids or sucralfate; omeprazole inhibits cyanocobalamin absorption

Distribution: Pts taking interacting meds or with low albumin states such as renal failure, and malnutrition may show evidence of toxicity despite normal serum levels, eg, nystagmus w phenytoin; warfarin displaced and therefore potentiated by allopurinol, metronidazole (Flagyl), Tm/S (Bactrim); phenytoin (Dilantin) potentiated by INH, benzodiazepines, phenothiazine; increase in plasma (α_1-acid glycoprotein leads to increased protein binding of basic drugs, thereby decreasing amount of free active drug, eg, lidocaine, and propanolol

Adipose tissue proportion increases from 18% to 36% (men) and from 36% to 48% (women); total body water decreases by 15% from ages 20 to 80 yr; therefore, increase in volume of distribution of lipophilic drugs, eg, sedative hypnotics, and decrease in hydrophilic drugs, eg, digoxin, aminoglycosides, penicillins

Excretion: Decrease in renal blood flow 1%/yr after age 50, GFR decreased by 35% between 3rd and 10th decades of life

Creatinine clearance (Creat Cl)
= [(140 − age) × weight in kg/serum creatinine × 72]
(× 0.85 if woman)

If < 30, cut the drug dose by half; digoxin toxicity not always recognized in the elderly so imperative to base dose on creatinine clear-

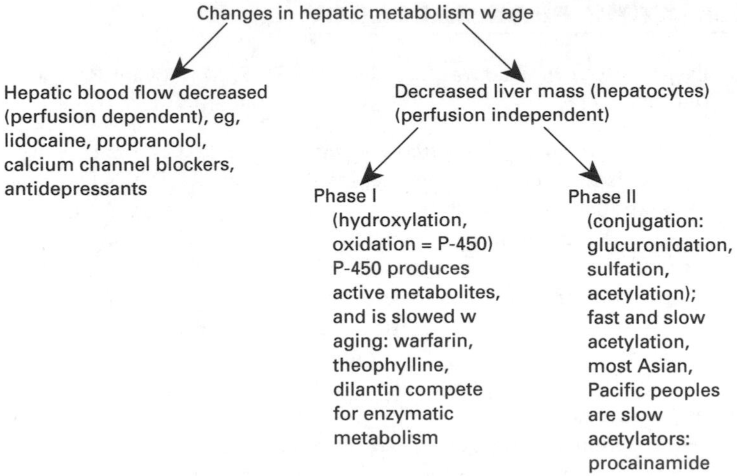

Changes in hepatic metabolism w age

Hepatic blood flow decreased (perfusion dependent), eg, lidocaine, propranolol, calcium channel blockers, antidepressants

Decreased liver mass (hepatocytes) (perfusion independent)

Phase I (hydroxylation, oxidation = P-450) P-450 produces active metabolites, and is slowed w aging: warfarin, theophylline, dilantin compete for enzymatic metabolism

Phase II (conjugation: glucuronidation, sulfation, acetylation); fast and slow acetylation, most Asian, Pacific peoples are slow acetylators: procainamide

Figure 1-1. Changes in hepatic metabolism with age.

ance (J Am Ger Soc 1996;44:54); can either lengthen drug interval or decrease drug dose (Drugs 1994;48:380):

Drug interval = (nl Creat Cl/pt's Creat Cl) × nl interval

Drug dose = (pt's Creat Cl/nl Creat Cl) × nl dose

Measured creatinine clearance may be better than estimated in higher-functioning elderly (J Am Ger Soc 1993;41:716); drug levels should be drawn just prior to scheduled dose after 3–5 half-lives of dosing

Metabolism: Drugs requiring phase 1 (oxidation, reduction, hydrolysis), eg, diazepam (Valium), lidocaine, isosorbide, are affected by decreased enzymatic activity of P-450 with aging; phase 2 (conjugation), eg, oxazepam (Serax), lorazepam (Ativan), metabolism is not affected by aging (Figure 1-1) (Med Let 1996;38:75)

More adverse drug interactions when renally excreted drugs used simultaneously, eg, digoxin not cleared when given with quinidine or verapamil; lithium not cleared when given with NSAIDs or thiazides; types of renal-drug interactions: (1) allergic is not dose-related and takes weeks to resolve, eg, methicillin, ACE inhibitors, NSAIDs, trimethoprim, cimetidine; (2) hemodynamic is dose-related and takes days to resolve, eg, anti-inflammatory drugs, ACE inhibitors; (3) toxic is dose-related and takes weeks to resolve, eg, gentamicin, phenacetin, lithium; (4) pseudoazotemia is dose-related and takes days to resolve, eg, trimethoprim, cimetidine (Am J Kidney Dis 1996;27:162)

Pharmacodynamics: Decreased receptor response: decreased effect of adrenergic medications, eg, β-adrenergic agonists, β-adrenergic blockers

Increased receptor response: increased effect of opiates, eg, morphine, and increased effect of benzodiazepines, eg, diazepam; clonazepin 0.5 mg hs and increase by 0.5 mg q 1–2 wk (drug half-life 48 h) and assess pt's gait; topical therapy: may add capsaicin cream 0.25%–0.75%, lower potency for first 2 wk then switch to higher potency, may tolerate better if applied w lidocaine ointment 2.5%–5.0% for first few days of treatment, may interfere with substance P (Life Sci 1979;25:1273), reduces tenderness and pain with only adverse effect of localized transient burning (J Rheum 1992;19:604; Ann IM 1994;121:133); consider neural blockade after all else fails

Pain (Management of cancer pain, U.S. Department of Health and Human Services Agency of Health Care Policy and Research;Storey P, Primer of palliative care, Academy of Hospice Phyicians; Pain, in Kemp C, Terminal illness, JB Lippincott, 1995:112)

Midrin, sumatriptan safer for migraines than ergots

Postherpetic neuralgia: constant pain: nortriptyline or desipramine 12.5–25.0 mg increased q 2–3 d in 10-mg increments as tolerated and if no benefit switch to nortriptyline or maprotiline and if still no benefit, add anticonvulsant; lancinating pain: carbamazepine 150 mg/d or alternative anticonvulsant may add antidepressant

Opioids for severe pain (Med Lett Drugs Ther 1993;35:1): morphine sulfate for cancer or postop pain: pain despite >12 mg/d, switch to 10 mg liquid morphine sulfate q 4 h with rescue dose (one-half regular q 4 h dose q 2–3 h); slow-release morphine q 12 h must be accompanied by immediate-release morphine for breakthrough pain (one-sixth to one-third of slow-release dose (sl, po, or pr); drowsiness occurs within first few hours of therapy, onset unlikely after this period; tolerance requires weeks to months of continuous administration, and may not develop at all in some pts; if no respiratory depression in 2–3 d of use, unlikely to develop, moni-

Table 1-2. Controversial Uses of Herbs

Potentially Beneficial Herbs	Potentially Dangerous Herbs
Chamomile: digestion	Chaparral: hepatitis
Echinacea: immunity booster	Comfrey: liver toxicity
Feverfew (0.2% parthenolide): migraine	Ephedra: raises BP, palpitations
Garlic: cholesterol	Lobela: acts like nicotine
Ginger: nausea, motion sickness	Yohimbine: weakness, nervous stimulation
Ginkgo biloba: helps w dementia (24% ginkgo flavone glycosides, 6% ginkgolides and bilobalide) 30–40 mg tid × 4–6 wk (Lancet 1992;340:1136)	
Hawthorn: HT and angina	
Mild thistle: liver damage	
Saw palmetto: enlarged prostate	
Valerian: mild sedating and tranquilizing effect	

From Shimonura SK, UCLA Intensive course in Geriatric Medicine and Board Review 1/96.

tor sleep respiratory rate, if does not fall below 12 breaths/min when dose increased, will not develop respiratory depression; physical or psychological dependence does not occur early in its administration; biphosphonates good adjuvant analgesic; pts get equally confused after the administration of epidural or general anesthesia (Jama 1995;274:44)

To convert oral narcotic to equivalent morphine sulfate po multiply by 0.15 for propoxyphene, 0.2 for meperidine, 0.3 for codeine, 0.5 for pentazocine, 2 for oxycodone, 3 for methadone, 8 for hydromorphone; to convert im narcotic to equivalent morphine sulfate po multiply by 1.5 for pentazocine, 6 for methadone, 40 for hydromorphone, 3 for morphine sulfate, 0.8 for meperidine, 30 for butorphanol (Ger Rev Syllabus 3rd ed 1996; p 179)

Management of Opioid-Induced Constipation (Nejm 1996;335: 1124): Prevention: 100 mg docusate sodium plus 17.2 mg sennosides po bid; 10 mg bisacodyl po hs if no bm in past 24 h, repeat in morning if no bm; titration: 100–200 mg docusate plus 34.4 mg sennosides po tid; 15 mg bisacodyl po tid; obstipation: 30–60 mL MOM + mineral oil 30 mL bid; 30–60 mL lactulose qid

Herbs: Table 1-2

Vitamins: 1–6 gm vit C reduces cold sx by 21% and shortens course by 1 d

Vitamin E boosts immune system response in elderly (Jama 1997; 277:1380)

Hormone Replacement Therapy (Nejm 1994;330:1062; Obgyn 1994;83: 161; J Am Ger Soc 1993;41:426; 1996;44:1): (also see pp 206– 208, osteoporosis, CAD)

  Estrogen: Conjugated 0.625 mg, or micronized estradiol 1.0 mg or estradiol valerate 1.0 mg or estropipate 0.625 mg or transdermal estradiol 0.05 or 5.0 qd plus cyclic medroxyprogesterone acetate 5.0–10.0 (d 1–12 or 1–14), or continuous w medroxyprogesterone acetate 2.5 or 5.0

  Evaluation of postmenopausal bleeding: Endometrial bx for bleeding, manage by switching to continuous-combined regimen, increase progesterone by 2.5 mg until amenorrhea or adverse effects occur, if sx persist >10 mo (28% of pts), then perform bx (Ann IM 1992;117:1038); if no atypia on bx specimen, increase progesterone, eg, 10mg/d for 14 d of the mo for 6 mo; if atypia present, dilatation and curettage indicated (Mayo Clin Proc 1995;70:803)

  25% of estrogen prescriptions remain unfilled

  Alternatives to Estrogen: Megestrol acetate (Megace), progestational agent, decreases hot flashes, (Nejm 1994;331:347; 1995; 332:1638,1889); micronized progesterone helps w insomnia (Med Clin N Am 1995;79:1337); phytoestrogens in high-soy diet of Japanese women associated w infrequent hot flashes and other menopausal sx (Lancet 1992;339:1233)

URINARY TRACT COLONIZATION/INFECTION

J Am Ger Soc 1996;44:927,1235; Clin Ger Med 1990;6:1; AIM 1990; 150:1389

Cause: *Escherichia coli* predominant pathogen (50%) in elderly; instrumentation and institutionalization lead to *Proteus mirabilis, Klebsiella* sp, *Enterobacter, Serratia,* and *Pseudomonas aeruginosa;* 25% of elderly with urinary catheters have enterococci in urine; coagulase-neg staphylococci in ambulatory elderly; resistant organisms, eg, *Citrobacter freundii, Providencia stuartii*

Epidem: F/M = 2:1; UTIs cause 30%–50% of all bacteremia and septicemia, catheter bacteriuria increases by 3%–10%/d; bacteriuria increased in NH (33%) secondary to immobility, DM, fecal/urinary incontinence, deteriorating mental status

Pathophys: Attachment of bacteria to epithelial cells of the bladder is promoted by the changing hormonal status of the elderly pt, BPH, prostatic or renal stone formation; and a decrease in bacteriostatic prostatic secretions, increased vaginal pH, decreased lactobacillus, anatomic weakening of pelvic floor; MS, DM, CVA, Alzheimer's cause impaired bladder emptying, bacterial colonization; fecal incontinence causes retrograde colonization

Sx: Dysuria, fever, urinary urgency, frequency, hematuria, suprapubic discomfort are UTI-specific sx; nonspecific sx of UTI much more frequent: eg, change in mental status, change in functional capacity, acute-onset incontinence, decreased appetite, weakness, falls, hypotension, abdominal pain, nausea and vomiting, increased blood sugar in diabetics; must have specific or nonspecific sx before beginning treatment

Si: Foul smelling urine more indicative of dehydration than UTI (NH Med 1997;5:101)

Crs:

Uncomplicated (first infection): Infrequent UTIs (separated by at least 2–3 mo), occurring in a functionally independent, community-based elder, with no hx of gu complications, improving within 24–48 h of beginning therapy

Complicated: Hospitalized pt, or recurrent UTIs (separated by 4 wk), recent instrumentation, or gu complications; relapsing infection (separated by 2 wk; bacterial persistence) less common, r/o stones, chronic prostatitis (positive UA after prostatic massage), pyelonephritis, and fistulas

Complc: Sepsis, chronic pyelonephritis

Lab: Clean-catch UA: combined pos reading for nitrates, leukocyte esterase highly predictive of a UTI, whether to culture if UA pos debatable; replace catheter to obtain fresh specimen

Xray: PVR, renal US if suspect chronic pyelonephritis, obstruction

Rx: Rx of asx bacteriuria not shown to decrease morbidity or mortality

Preventive: Only catheterize when:
1. Retention unmanageable surgically
2. Risk of wound infection from incontinence high
3. Terminally ill pt w pain on movement and change of clothes
4. Pt preference when not responding to other incontinence therapy
5. Bacteriuria 48 h after short-term catheter: rx as sx UTI

Cranberry juice 300 mL/d × 6 mo (Jama 1994;271:751), 2 gm vit C

Suppress recurrent infections (>3/yr) or w h/o urosepsis: Tm/S (1 tab qd in M and one-half tab in F), and continue as long as UA neg, may use nitrofurantoin in this setting as well; intravaginal estrogen decreases pH, reducing colonization w gram-neg bacilli (Nejm 1993;329:753), long-term daily cranberry juice (Jama 1994;271:751)

Therapeutic: Treat symptomatic bacteriuria × 7 d in F, 14 d in M; rx nonspecific sxs at their first occurrence; if they do not respond to rx, sx may not be indicative of UTI; rx asymptomatic bacteriuria in pts with h/o short-term catheters, urinary manipulation, and instrumentation (Arch IM 1990;150:1389)

- Uncomplicated: Tm/S or amoxicillin, if resistance is suspected or drug allergy exists, use a quinolone (ciprofloxacin)
- Complicated: Stable outpatient or NH pt: start with a quinolone and change to narrower-spectrum drug once sensitivities have returned, × 14 d for T° >101 for upper UTI

Unstable (pt, NH pt): ampicillin and ceftriaxone im q 12–24 h in NH, remove and replace catheters; (hospitalized pt): ampicillin and gentamycin IV, vancomycin and gentamycin IV, fluoroquinolones and ampicillin IV, 3rd generation cephalosporin or aztreonam IV (NH Med 1997;5:100); Chronic bacterial prostatitis: Tm/S or quinolone × 4 wk

CONSTIPATION

Mayo Clin Proc 1996;71:81; J Am Ger Soc 1993;41:1130; Geriatrics 1989;44:53; J Am Ger Soc 1994;42:701

Cause:

Primary Causes: Decrease in large-bowel motility due to decreased fiber, decreased fluid, immobility, laxative abuse

Secondary Causes: Aluminum- or Fe-containing meds, anticholinergics, calcium channel blockers (verapamil), antipsychotics, diuretics, narcotics, antiparkinsonian medications, colonic-anorectal disorders (diverticula, irritable bowel, megacolon, hemorrhoids, strictures, polyps, colorectal cancer), DM, hypothyroidism, hyper/hypoparathyroidism, CNS central lesions, Parkinson's,

CVA, dementia, hypokalemia, hypercalcemia (decreased neural conduction time), depression and dementia also associated with constipation

Epidem: Subjective nature of the complaint makes accurate determination of the prevalence of true constipation difficult; 10% for those >75 (Gerontol Clin 1972;14:56), 30%–50% of elders use laxatives regularly

Pathophys:
  Definitions:
  - Functional constipation: straining >25% of time, or hard stools >25% of time, or feeling of incomplete evacuation >25% of time, <3 bms/wk
  - Rectal outlet delay (prolonged defecation secondary to anorectal dysfunction): anal blockage and prolonged defecation, or manual disimpaction needed (Gastroenterol Int 1991;4:99)

  Frail/institutionalized pts w increased total gut transit time develop colonic dilatation due to decrease in intraluminal pressures; increased gut transit time also caused by a disruption in coordinated segmental motion of the colonic circular smooth muscle, impaired rectal sensation and tone; also rectal dyschezia or increased rectal tone (irritable bowel syndrome); weakening of abdominal muscles and decreased external and internal anal sphincter tone

Sx: Change in usual bowel frequency less than 3 bms/wk, straining with evacuation and prolonged defecation (10 min or more for completion of bm), fecal soiling and/or fecal incontinence; abdominal distension and discomfort, and the need for manual disimpaction

Si: Diminished bowel sounds; lax abdominal musculature; masses in sigmoid, transverse, and descending colon; decreased rectal tone; decreased perianal sensation and anal reflex; presence of hard stool in rectal vault (empty vault common and does not preclude a high impaction); soft stool impacted in rectal vault may indicate rectal dysfunction; masses; hemorrhoids; fissures; oozing stool (overflow diarrhea), distended abdomen, nausea/vomiting, hard stool in rectum or colon; chronic or semiacute dehydration with tenting of sternal skin

Crs: May be chronic or acute; r/o irritable bowel syndrome (usually associated with a long hx of bowel disorders, "gas problems," abdominal pain relieved by defecation, and alternation between constipation and diarrhea); colorectal cancer and obstruction, anal fissure, rectal ischemia, and anorectal tumor may be associated with rectal pain on defecation

Cmplc: Cardiovascular (angina, MI, arrhythmias); megacolon (volvulus of sigmoid, cecal rupture); rectal prolapse; fecal incontinence (UTIs and sepsis, decubitus ulcers); hemorrhoids; laxative abuse

Lab: Fasting glucose, TSH (r/o hypothyroidism), hypercalcemia, hypokalemia, BUN, creatinine, guaiac stool, urine specific gravity

Xray: Flat plate of abdomen to r/o impaction; barium studies not recommended due to barium retention; colonoscopy if colonic cancer is suspected (anemia, family hx, or guaiac-pos stools) (Mayo Clin Proc 1996;71:81)

Rx:

Preventive: Increase fluid intake to 1200–2000 mL/d; then increase fiber intake (dietary fiber or OTC supplements, eg, Citrucel)—must take at least 1200 mL fluid/d if using fiber supplementation; begin regular exercise program; adjust toileting schedule to coincide with natural urge to defecate; consider morning coffee or tea; avoid meds that lead to constipation; avoid routine use of stimulant laxatives

Therapeutic: Initiate preventive regime, as above; increase fiber (Citrucel), 1 tsp up to tid is helpful except if pt is bedridden, has <1000 mL fluid intake/d, or has a hx of megacolon or volvulus

For slow transit: use laxatives in increasing order of strength as follows: sorbitol 15–30 mL qd to tid; MOM 15–30 mL qd or bid—contraindicated in moderate renal insufficiency; senna, 30 mg q h 3× wk (for maintenance); bisacodyl 10 mg supplement up to 3× wk; for rectal dyschezia: glycerin supplement 3× wk or up to qd; tap water enema, 500 mL/rectum as needed; mineral oil enema 100–250 mL qd

For fecal impaction: digital disimpaction followed by oil retention enemas and subsequent tap water enemas qd until clear; follow with cathartics to cleanse colon; senna 30 mg up to tid and sorbitol 30 mL up to tid; if large fecal load still present (but without obstruction, give 1–2 L polyethylene glycol (Go-lytely)

When abdominal xray is clear of impaction, begin maintenance bowel regime as above; stool softeners (docusate sodium (Colace)) only when straining is to be avoided (post-MI, angina, hemorrhoids, postsurgery), always avoid use of highly irritant laxatives, such as phenolphthalein (Ex-Lax, Correctol)

Team Management: Nursing staff, family assist pt to upright commode when urge to defecate occurs; osteopathic maneuvers: sacral rocking (gentle pressure on sacrum w inspiration while pt prone)

MALNUTRITION

Nurs Home Med 1994;2:206; Geriatrics 1990;45:7; Reuben D, Nutritional problems and assessment, UCLA intensive geriatric review course, 1/19/96; J Am Ger Soc 1995;43:415; Ger Rev Syllabus 3rd ed 1996, 145–151

Cause: Inadequate intake, inadequate dentition, poverty and inadequate range of food groups, malabsorption, nutrient-drug interactions, chronic disease, or acute insult; taste decreased secondary to decreased olfaction w age (J Gerontol 1986;41:460)
Dehydration: reduced access to fluids, decreased thirst perception, reduced response to serum osmolality, decreased ability to concentrate urine following fluid deprivation

Epidem: Malnutrition occurs in 37%–40% of community elderly, 35%–65% of hospitalized elderly, 19%–58% of institutionalized elderly (Nurs Home Med 1994;2:206)

Sx: Nutritional hx from the pt or caregiver regarding eating preferences, restrictions, and allergies; use of mineral/vit supplements, and non-prescription meds; taste change, chewing, swallowing problems, nausea/vomiting/diarrhea

Si: D-E-N-T-A-L Screening Survey (J Am Ger Soc 1996;44:980):
Dry mouth
Eating difficulty
No recent dental care
Tooth or mouth pain
Alteration or change in food selection
Lesions, sores, or lumps in the mouth
Changes seen in nutritional deficiencies may be mistaken for changes occurring with aging on screening exam (brittle hair and nails, sunken eyes, pale sclerae, prominence of the bony skeleton, especially the extremities and chest cavity); may also see cracked lips, sores around the mouth, poor dentition, magenta tongue, muscle wasting, peripheral edema, blunted mental status

Height and weight most reliable of the anthropomorphic measurements; assess ability to self-feed; when intake is difficult to assess or is obviously poor, obtain a 24–72-h calorie count (in *NH* 2 wk after admission, allowing the pt to settle into environment)

Meds that interfere w vits:

Trimethoprim and phenytoin interfere w folate

Cholestyramine, mineral oil, and neomycin interfere w vit A absorption (night blindness)

Hydralazine is a vit B_6 antagonist; INH increases vit B_6 urinary excretion

Lab: Assess the severity of weight loss by determining the ratio of the pt's ABW to IBW; for M calculated at 106 pounds for the first 5 feet and 6 pounds for each inch above 5 feet; for F it is 100 pounds for the first 5 feet and 5 pounds for each inch above 5 feet

Knee height measurements, arm span, or summation of body parts may be used to accurately assess height in pts who are unable to stand erect (Gottschlich M, Matavese L, Shronts EP, eds, Nutrition support dietetics core curriculum, 2nd ed, Silver Spring, MD, American Society of Parenteral and Enteral Nutrition, 1993:44); take into account ethnic variation and compare to other family members; ABW is affected by hydration status and therefore dehydration should be r/o before other causes of weight loss are investigated

Significant weight loss: 2% in 1 wk or 5% in 1 mo; 7.5% in 3 mo; 10% decrease in weight from the UBW in 6 mo

Crs: Vits B_1, C become deficient over wk to mo while fat-soluble vits (A<D<E<K) take longer because of enterohepatic circulation; obesity about the waist and abdomen increases free fatty acids in the portal system leading to increased lipid production and CAD

Complc: Pressure sore formation, compromised immune function, increased rate of infection, longer recuperation periods, and consequent loss of independence

Rx:

Prevention: Older pts trying to gain weight require 30–35 kcal/kg IBW; check lytes prior to aggressive nutritional support; if tube feeding indicated, start at 20 kcal/kg IBW and slowly advance to 30–35 kcal/kg IBW; energy needs for pts whose weight is <76% of IBW should be calculated using ABW, not IBW which could result in an overestimate of caloric requirements, extreme fluid, lyte shifts

Estimate protein needs using albumin levels; albumin has half-life of 21 d, reflects previous protein expenditure due to a number of causes, eg, liver disease, infection, nephrotic syndrome, postop states, inadequate intake and malabsorption; dehydration may falsely elevate albumin; albumin levels of 3.1–3.5 gm/dL indicate mild depletion; 2.6–3.1 gm/dL moderate depletion; and <2.6 gm/dL severe depletion; low albumin a predictor of mortality as well (Jama 1994;272:1036); single best predictor of death in malnourished NH pt is cholesterol below 150 mg/dL (J Am Ger Soc 1996;44:37)

NH pts require 1 gm/kg IBW/d of protein; this increases to 1.2 gm/kg IBW in presence of infection or pressure sores, and to 1.5 gm/kg IBW with overwhelming infection and after major surgery; protein provides 20% of the energy from regular diet, therefore 1800-cal diet furnishes 90 gm of protein; most dietary supplements provide 10 gm of protein/can (240 mL)

Restrictive diets: 3 gm Na, ADA diet not likely to improve the status of CHF or DM in old-old, more likely to cause protein-energy malnutrition

Supplemental diets: poor wound healing, consider vit C 500 mg/d and zinc sulfate 220 mg tid (Ann IM 1988;109:890)

Treatment: Of dehydration: fluid requirements of 1500 mL/d;

Hypernatremia: require 30 mL free water/kg body weight, or replace 25%–30% of deficit/d:

Free water deficit = 0.6 × IBW

× (1 − 140/measured serum Na)

(Nejm 1977;297:1444)

Hypodermoclysis: sc fluids when iv access difficult, for acute illness (Jama 1995;274:1552; J Am Ger Soc 1996;44:969)

Vitamin supplementation: low-dose multivitamin enhances lymphocyte proliferation, IL-2 production, decreases infection risk in elderly

• W aging skin vit D synthesis from sunlight decreased, therefore supplement those at risk for osteoporosis, especially important in institutionalized elderly; vit K also helps w bone metabolism

• Vit B_6 helps maintain glucose tolerance, cognitive function, enhances aging immune system, but decreases the effectiveness of L-dopa in treatment of Parkinson's

• Vit B_{12} protects against high homocysteine levels associated w stroke, neither vit B_{12} nor folic acid absorbed well in atrophic gastritis, screen for vit B_{12} deficiency (J Am Ger Soc 1995;43: 1290), oral B_{12} (1000–2000 µgm/d) effective in absence of intrinsic factor

- Increased consumption of leafy vegetables rich in retinoids decreases risk of age-related macular degeneration (Jama 1994; 272:1413)
- Antioxidant vits C, E, and β-carotene may reduce risk of cancer, cataracts, and heart disease (Nutr Rev 1994:52:S15) vs β-carotenes not shown to help (Nejm 1996;334:1145,1150)
  Fiber: psyllium-containing products also lower cholesterol when given w meals, phytate (cereals, legumes, vegetables) can impair calcium, zinc absorption

VISION

CATARACTS

UCLA intensive geriatric review course, 1/96; Ger Rev Syllabus 3rd ed, 1996, p 138–144

Cause: Sun exposure, age, trauma, uveitis, retinitis pigmentosa, intraocular malignancies, DM, hypoparathyroidism, hypothyroidism, steroids (topical as well as systemic), congenital, environmental/UV radiation, smoking, ?diets low in antioxidants

Epidem: 18% of those age 65–74 yr and 46% age >75 yr; leading cause of reversible blindness in the U.S., second leading cause of overall blindness in the U.S., cataract extraction is the most frequently performed surgical intervention on the Medicare population (12% of the 1995 Medicare budget)

Pathophys: Water-insoluble proteins increase w age, leading to brown pigmentation of lens:

- Nuclear cataract (most common): sclerosis of fibers in the lens w increased refractive index secondary to color changes
- Anterior subcapsular: usually iritis leads to adherence to the lens, forming posterior synechiae and eventually, w epithelial cell proliferation, a subcapsular connective tissue plaque; lens is opaci-fied and liquified until the entire lens cortex is involved, forming a "mature" cataract

- Posterior subcapsular: formed by epithelial cells that migrate beneath the posterior capsule and enlarge

Sx: Reduced visual acuity although may report improved near vision (nuclear), distant or increased glare (posterior subcapsular)

Si: Opacities often visible on ophthalmoscopic exam; difficult to visualize fundus

Crs: Develop after age 40, almost anyone who lives long enough will develop them; painless progressive variable loss of vision

Cmplc: R/o normal changes of aging: dark adaptation, decreased peripheral vision, diminished perception of low-contrast objects; advanced cataract may swell and the capsule may become leaky, leaking into the anterior chamber causing secondary glaucoma

Rx:

- 90% of extractions are extracapsular, leaving the posterior capsule in place, providing an anchor for the intraocular lens
- Phacoemulsification (ultrasonic wave) used to pulverize the lens so it can be aspirated prior to placement of implant, less valuable for pts w hard sclerotic nuclear cataracts
- Lens replaced by eyeglass, contact lens, or preferably, implant
- Complications of treatment: opacification of posterior capsule (50% over 3-yr period)—can use laser to correct this w improvement in 90% of pts
- Pts w macular degeneration, also related to sun exposure, may also have cataracts; therefore do not repair cataracts when there is coexistent severe macular degeneration (sometimes difficult clinical decision)
- Complication rates of surgery low: faulty wound closure w aqueous humor leakage and intractable secondary glaucoma, explosive choroidal hemorrhage which can cause blindness, endophthalmitis requiring hopitalization for iv antibiotics and corticosteroids (Merck manual of geriatrics, 1995)

GLAUCOMA

Cause: Primary open-angle glaucoma (POAG): 70% of cases due to impaired aqueous drainage through the trabecular meshwork; POAG accounts for 90% of glaucoma in the elderly in the U.S.; narrow-angle (NAG): steroid-induced, traumatic, inflammatory, neovascular, low tension

Epidem: Risk factors: increased age, females; weaker association with HT, cardiovascular disease, diabetes, smoking, UV light exposure, and diet; POAG: 6× more common in blacks whereas NAG more prevalent among Orientals, especially Chinese

Pathophys: POAG: anatomically normal outflow channels but increased resistance to aqueous humor outflow from gradual meshwork occlusion.

NAG: as lens thickens, anterior chamber is made more shallow, especially in farsighted pts w smaller eyes; elevated intraocular pressure occurs when the base of the iris is pushed forward, sealing off trabecular meshwork outflow; aqueous humor continuously produced by the eye circulating through the anterior chamber cannot leave through outflow channels, producing intraocular pressure of 50–60 mmHg in hours (nl intraocular pressure = 20 mmHg), irreversible changes in 48–72 h

Crs: POAG: 2% visual field loss/yr (Nejm 1993;328:1097)

Sx: POAG: asx till very late, gradual loss of visual fields over years; NAG: acute pain, blurred vision, halos from corneal edema, nausea

Si: POAG: diagnosis depends on the presence of optic nerve excavation (cupping), visual field defects, w or w/o intraocular pressure elevation (common but not a diagnostic feature); if intraocular pressure <21 mmHg but no visual field deficit, then only ocular HT

Rx:

POAG:

Preventive: Yearly intraocular pressure measurement w Shiøtz tonometer and ophthalmoscopic exam for optic head excavation increases detection rate to 80%, usually done by optometrist or ophthalmologist; stereoscopic equipment and formal visual field testing increase the accuracy of diagnosis

Therapeutic: Management falls largely to ophthalmologist and is directed toward lowering intraocular pressure (does not always stop progression of visual loss):

Topical:
- β-Blockers reduce the secretion of aqueous humor, watch for systemic side effects of β-blockers (bradycardia, CHF)
- Adrenergics, eg, epinephrine decreases aqueous humor production and increases its outflow through the trabecular meshwork
- Miotics, eg, pilocarpine, carbachol constrict pupil-stimulating longitudinal muscle fibers of the ciliary body, thereby opening the trabecular meshwork pores

Oral:
- Carbonic anhydrase inhibitors, eg, acetazolamide decreases production of aqueous humor, numerous adverse effects in the elderly—confusion, paresthesias, drowsiness, anorexia, calcium phosphate renal stones

Surgical (filtration procedures designed to create drainage between the anterior chamber and the subconjunctival space) Follow q 6 mo

NAG: Emergency pilocarpine 2%–4% q 5 min × 6, or acetazolamide 250 mg

Surgical: laser iridotomy within 24 h, expect cure

MACULAR DEGENERATION

UCLA intensive geriatric review course, 1/96

Cause:

Epidem: The leading cause of irreversible blindness in U.S. elderly; among people >55 yr in the U.S., 2.2% are blind in one eye from macular degeneration; increased w age, whites, females; weaker association with HT, cardiovascular disease, diabetes, smoking (Jama 1996;276:1141,1147), UV light exposure

Pathophys: Degenerative changes in the macula lead to loss of fine central vision, but not peripheral vision; since macular changes such as pigment mottling and the appearance of drusen also occur in all older retinae, the label of acute macular degeneration is only used when there is accompanying loss of visual acuity; for both of these conditions the anatomic changes lie on a continuum; therefore the criteria for defining a diseased vs healthy eye in an older person is difficult

Sx: Sudden or recent central vision loss, blurred vision, distortion, new scotomata indicate neovascularization; Amsler grid facilitates monitoring

Si: Hard yellow-white pinhead-size drusen; localized disorder of retinal pigmented epithelium vs soft drusen more widespread damage; 3 forms: dry or atrophic (80%–90% w central loss of vision), subretinal neovascular membrane, retinal pigment epithelial detachment with drusen

Rx:

- Low vision aids: magnifying devices, eg, magnified TV, special lighting (J Am Optom Assoc 1988;59:307; Geriatrics 1995; 50(12):51)
- Photocoagulation (Arch Ophthalmol 1994;112:489): indicated for symptomatic choroidal neovascularization outside foveal avascular zone (minority of pts), postpones visual loss; complc: scar if "runoff" beyond intended area of treatment

Team Management: Low vision aids, support group

DIABETIC RETINOPATHY

Cause: Diabetes neovascularization and hemorrhage

Epidem: 3rd leading cause of adult blindness (7% of all blindness); increased prevalence (3%) with greater longevity, positively correlated with the duration of diabetes

Pathophys: Selective loss of mural cells in the basement membrane of retinal capillaries; when glucose is converted by aldose reductase to sorbitol, water moves into the mural cells and they rupture; mural cells have contractile properties, and therefore their loss results in capillary dilatation, leading to increased volume of blood flow and resultant microaneurysms, which hemorrhage and lead to exudate formation

Sx: Loss of vision, glaucoma in end stages

Si:

Nonproliferative: Hemorrhages in both the nerve fiber and mid retinal layers, cotton wool spots (nerve fiber layer infarcts), vascular dilatation and tortuousness, microaneurysms, macular edema

> **Proliferative:** Neovascularization at the disc and, elsewhere, preretinal/vitreous hemorrhage, traction retinal detachment, posterior retinal breaks, glaucoma, macular edema

Crs: Early 3–5 yr first see minimal visual loss from macular edema, or clouding of vision from small vitreous hemorrhage, microaneurysms (>5 in each eye); then nonproliferative changes; then proliferative changes

Rx:

> **Preventive:** Annual ophthalmologic exam; ? correlation between ACE inhibitor and postponement of diabetic retinopathy (Am J Med Sci 1993;305:280); tight diabetic control reduces progression
>
> **Therapeutic:** Aldose reductase inhibitor, Epalrestat, to decrease sorbitol; proliferative: laser photocoagulation early slows down visual loss; ? w nonproliferative, ?vitrectomy w impending retinal detachment

HEARING PROBLEMS

UCLA intensive geriatric review course, 1/96

Cause:

- Sensorineural (most common): cochlea or auditory nerve damage due to loud noise (usually bilateral); ototoxic drug effects may be delayed in onset; aminoglycosides dose-related less common than vestibular disturbance and tinnitus; vestibular disturbance and tinnitus are often first signs, taking as much as 2 wk to abate after drug discontinued; aging (presbycusis: high-frequency loss); unilateral causes include trauma, infection, acoustic neuroma, Meniere's—also associated w peripheral vertigo
- Conductive (uncommon): cerumen impaction, middle ear disease, otosclerosis
- Central hearing loss: impaired speech discrimination beyond what would be expected based on threshold loss (10% of cognitively impaired)

Epidem: Prevalence increases with age; in the Framingham cohort 41%

>65 yr had some level of impairment, only 10% had tried hearing aids; 80% of men between 85 and 90 yr reported having trouble hearing; in NHs prevalence ranges from 50%–100%

Si: Whisper test from behind pt; observation of lip-reading ("intentness index"); types of hearing loss:
- Conductive: bone thresholds > air thresholds
- Sensorineural: both air and bone thresholds are elevated

Crs: Declines 2× faster in men than women; women have more sensitive hearing above 1000-Hz frequency, while men have more sensitive hearing at lower frequencies (J Acoust Soc Am 1995;97:1196)

Cmplc: Social isolation/withdrawal from conversations, frustration/resentment, mislabeled with dementia, depression, greater risk of falling, impaired mobility, cognitive impairment

Lab: Audiometry tests and interpretation: measured in decibels at which the stimulus can be heard 50% of the time, test ability to understand words (speech discrimination)

Rx:

Conductive:
- Amplification: improvement in social function, emotional well-being, communication function, less depression; hearing aids are most helpful for understanding speech, and listening to TV or movies, not as helpful in crowded or noisy situations; barriers: cost (largest obstacle, $700–$1000), self-perceived handicap, difficulties with the small controls due to arthritis, excessive feedback from ear-mold fittings; if loss >80 dB, only limited improvement w hearing aid
- Involvement of a hearing aid specialist for identification of appropriate equipment and training and counseling; adjustment may take weeks to months and is strongly influenced by motivation

Team Management: Physician-patient relationship: minimize background noise as much as possible, use good lighting, face the person at eye level, encourage pts to wear their hearing aids to an office visit, speak clearly from closer range, and lower pitch if possible rather than shouting, use gestures and write down important instructions

INCONTINENCE

URGE INCONTINENCE

AHCPR Publc No. 92-0039, US Pub Hlth Svc, 1992; Nejm 1989;320:1; 1985;313:800; Lancet 1995;346:94; Ann IM 1995;122:438

Cause: Decreased CNS inhibition common in many normal elders, accentuated in dementia (voiding dysfunction in NPH results from paraventricular compression of frontal inhibitory centers leading to urge incontinence), Parkinson's, CVA, or cervical stenosis; or with parasympathomimetic drugs like bethanechol (Urecholine), cisapride; or irritation from cystitis, prostatitis, BPH, bladder tumor

Epidem: One-third have urge incontinence (common in community-dwelling elderly)

Pathophys: Detrusor overactivity may be due to CNS lesion, detrusor hyperreflexia, or aging (detrusor instability) (Urol Clin N Am 1996;23:55)

Detrusor instability w (most common form in the elderly) (J Urol 1993;150:1668) or w/o impaired contractility

Sx: Moments warning, volume of urine lost may be large or small; stained clothing

Lab: Cystometrics show spastic contractions

Rx:

- Antibiotics for any infection
- If minimal in community-dwelling elderly: planned voiding, avoid caffeine, alcohol, carbonated drinks
- Biofeedback (Ann IM 1985;103:507), pelvic exercises, extend voiding intervals by half-hour increments once dry (JAMA 1991;265:609); prompted voiding q 2 h helps cognitively impaired pts (J Am Ger Soc 1990;38:356) and is 25%–40% effective (Dis Mo 1992;38:65)
- Oxybutynin (Ditropan) 5 mg po tid (anticholinergics, ie, parasympathetic inhibition), adding oxybutynin to prompted voiding more effective (J Am Ger Soc 1995;43:610), or propantheline 7.5–30.0 mg po tid
- Imipramine 25–50 mg po hs (α-stimulation, parasympathetic inhibition)
- Flavoxate not effective

- Trial of bladder relaxants; if urinary retention >150 mL, suspect detrusor hyperreflexia coexisting w mild urinary outflow obstruction in males, or detrusor overactivity w impaired contractility; in pts w detrusor hyperreflexia and impaired contractility in which involuntary contractions are only provoked at higher bladder volumes, catheterize hs; avoid bladder relaxants (Jama 1996;267:1832)
- Estrogen may be useful in women w urge incontinence, also ameliorates dyspareunia and reduces the frequency of recurrent cystitis (Nejm 1993;329:753)
- Refer for further urologic w/u if recurrent UTIs (Ann IM 1995;122: 749), microscopic hematuria, failure to respond to pharmacologic or behavoral treatment, diagnostic uncertainty

OVERFLOW INCONTINENCE

Cause: Bladder outlet obstruction, eg, BPH, uterine prolapse, large cystocele, ureteral stenosis (associated w atrophic vaginitis), constipation (up to 10% in hospitalized pts), α-stimulant drugs, neuropathy (impaired sensory input to sacral micturition center); or diminished detrusor strength (flaccid due to lower motor neuron disease); or herpes zoster (from pain); or neurosyphilis which causes detrusor sphincter dyssynergy (Urol Clin N Am 1996;23: 11); or meds like anticholinergics, calcium channel blockers, smooth muscle relaxants, opiates

Epidem: Overflow incontinence less common than other forms of incontinence

Sx: Obstructive w diminished urinary stream, leakage of urine usually small amounts, frequency; if neuropathic, will have no sensation of bladder fullness

Si: Prostate's palpated size correlates poorly w actual size; suprapubic and abdominal exam for distended bladder

Lab: PVR >200 mL (easy office procedure); in women w large cystoceles, urine may "puddle" below catheter's reach, giving falsely low value for PVR; obtain renal function tests (Ouslander 1996, UCLA Intensive Geriatric Review Course, 1/96), and refer for cystometrics or voiding cystourethrogram; cystometrics show no contractions w 400+ mL when due to diminished sensation

Rx:

- Stool softeners for constipation
- Rx prolapse or BPH, finasteride modest and delayed benefits (Nejm 1992;327:1185), less extensive resection of prostate w local anesthesia in frail elderly men
- Block sphincter constriction (α-blockade) w prazosin (Minipress) 1–2 mg po tid or terazosin (Hytrin); finasteride (5α-reductase inhibitor decreases BPH) not as effective (Ann IM 1995;122:438)
- Bladder neuropathy from cobalamin deficiency reversible w vit B_{12} replacement (J Intern Med 1992;231:313); 60% of diabetics w incontinence do not have neuropathic bladder, they have constipation from autonomic neuropathy (J Am Ger Soc 1993;41:1130)
- Self-catheterization (J Am Ger Soc 1990;38:364) may be impractical in frail elderly (Ouslander 1996, UCLA Intensive Geriatric Review Course, 1/96); long-term catheters indicated in 1%–2% pts
- Increase detrusor strength w bethanechol (Urecholine) 10+ mg po tid, mostly useful in the setting of anticholinergic agents that can't be discontinued, or phenoxybenzamine (Dibenzyline) 10 mg po qd (parasympathomimetics); monitor PVR
- Wood pulp–containing absorbent undergarments superior to polymer gel; garments for women and men differ because different target zone of urinary loss (Urol Clin N Am 1996;23:11)
- Indwelling catheter care: do not irrigate or clamp; leakage may be due to bladder spasm; therefore use smaller catheter; treat only symptomatic UTIs and do not use prophylaxis; consider acidification if no urea-splitting organisms and silicon catheter if obstruction occurs frequently
- Refer for urologic w/u if large cystourethrocele, markedly enlarged prostate (check PSA first), symptoms or signs of obstruction, and pt is a surgical candidate

STRESS INCONTINENCE

Cause: Estrogen deficiency effect on urethral mucosa; or pelvic relaxation after childbirth or urologic surgery; neuropathies; α-blocking meds

Epidem: One-third have mixed stress and urge incontinence

Pathophys: Sphincter insufficiency

Sx: Loss of urine w cough, sneeze, laugh

Si: Cystocele on physical exam if due to pelvic relaxation

Lab:

- Voiding record kept for 48–72 h useful: milder form of intrinsic sphincter deficiency occurs in older women resulting from urethral atrophy; they leak urine at higher amounts of bladder capacity (200 mL); therefore, if incontinent in morning after full night's sleep, then probably have volume-dependent stress incontinence
- Urinary stress test: pt should tolerate 300–500 mL before becoming very uncomfortable; if tolerates <250 mL, need further evaluation for interstitial cystitis (pain related to voiding without objective evidence of disease, which may be due to deficiency in bladder lining, autoimmune phenomena, r/o carcinoma-in-situ w cystoscopy) (Waxman J, Texas A+M Univ Health Science Ctr, Conference on women's health, 2/28/96, Cancun, Mexico)

Rx:

- Kegel exercises 20–200 daily (J Gerontol 1993;48:M167); postural maneuvers (Obgyn 1994;84:770); vaginal weights better than Kegels; pesaries (J Am Ger Soc 1992;40:635)
- Estrogen: start w oral estrogen unless worried about breast cancer risk, in which case can take intermittently po or try vaginal administration 0.5–1.0 gm of Premarin cream 1–2 mo, then taper; most can be weaned to 2–4×/mo (Urol Clin N Am 1996;23:55); if chronic therapy necessary, consider adding progestational agent in pts who still have a uterus; need to treat concurrently w α-agonist or exercises to be effective (Ouslander 1996, UCLA Intensive Geriatric Review Course, 1/96)
- Of neuropathic types, imipramine 25+ mg hs (α-stimulation, parasympathetic inhibition) or phenylpropanolamine 25–75 mg bid (α-stimulation); or biofeedback (Ann IM 1985;103:507)
- Surgery (bladder neck suspension safe and effective, AP repair, sphincter repairs)

FUNCTIONAL INCONTINENCE

Cause: Can't get to toilet

Si: All normal

Rx: Schedules plus reinforcement of prompted voiding w 25%–40% response rate can be identified during a 3-d trial period (Jama 1995;273:1366)

FEMALE SEXUAL DYSFUNCTION

Cause: Uterus not necessary for orgasm; radical procedures to remove part of the vagina do not affect ability to have orgasm (Obgyn 1993;81:357); quality of first sexual experience after breast cancer treatment strongly influences later sexual development (CA 1988; 38:154); women receive less sexual counseling after acute MI than do men; in couples who do not resume sexual activity there is deterioration of their emotional relationships (Heart Lung 1987;16: 154); any major illness in self or partner can become "watershed point"

Epidem: Young people, especially physicians, underrate the extent of sexual interest of older people

Pathophys: Androgens derived largely from the adrenal gland and a small amount from the ovaries sustain libido; however, coital activity is not correlated w blood levels of estradiol, testosterone, androstenedione, FSH, or LH (Maturitas 1991;13:43)

Sx: Key screening questions: Are you sexually active? Do you have a healthy partner? Is there a change in your level of desire? Is there any discomfort w sexual activity? Is vaginal dryness a problem? Is there difficulty achieving orgasm?; dyspareunia (in one-third of women >65 yr) associated w postmenopausal urogenital atrophy including a feeling of dryness, tightness, vaginal irritation, burning w coitus, and postcoital spotting and soreness; w very old, explore from perspective of sexual feelings, thoughts, always ask about self-stimulation, masturbation (at least once in establishing relationship with pt); can be useful to start with "Sexual feelings continue to be important for many people during aging—this can sometimes surprise people as they get older—how would you describe this part of you?"

Si: Look for signs of vaginitis (erythema introitus), atrophy (thinned, pallorous mucosa), depression

Crs: Single most significant determinant of sexual activity is unavailability of partner; rate of sexual activity earlier in life persists into old age; orgasm usually survives most illness and treatments; sexual touching almost always continues to be pleasurable; most couples resume sexual activity 7 mo after acute MI; risk of death during sexual intercourse very low

Rx:

Prevention: Important to let older women know that sexual fantasies, desires are normal, but be nonjudgmental about those who are satisfied w abstinence; open discussion of body image w couples (after breast removal, w placement of ostomy bags, incontinence, stroke); assumption of heterosexuality leads to a reluctance of older lesbians to interact w health system (J Gerontol Nurs 1990;16:35); staff attitudes and beliefs central problem for NH elderly who are categorized as having sexual problems (J Am Ger Soc 1987:35:331; Arch Sex Behav 1994;23:231); β-blocking agents decrease vaginal lubrication; ACE inhibitors and calcium channel blockers do not cause sexual dysfunction; all psychotropic drugs associated w inhibition of sexual function; antidepressants can cause anorgasmia (J Clin Psychiatry 1991;52:66); alcohol causes sexual dysfunction, though very small amounts may help some people

Therapeutic: Formal sex education yields more permissive attitudes (Int J Aging Hum Dev 1982;15:121); estrogen therapy reverses atrophic changes but may take as long as 6–12 mo; water-based lubricants better, eg, Astroglide, Replens; vaginismus (involuntary vaginal muscle contractions because of painful intercourse) responds to estrogen and voluntary contraction and relaxation of introitus w finger in the introitus, then w partner penetration in stages; androgen controversial (give progestational agent to avoid endometrial hyperplasia); masturbation (manual or w mechanical device); recommended reading for pts: Gershenfeld M, How to find love and sex and intimacy after age 50: a woman's guide, Ballantine, 1991; Silverstone B, Growing older together: a couple's guide to understanding and coping w the challenges of later life, Pantheon, 1992

MALE SEXUAL DYSFUNCTION (IMPOTENCE)

J Am Ger Soc 1987;35:1015; 1988;36:57; Arch IM 1989;149: 1365; Ger Rev Syllabus 3rd ed., 1996, p. 310–312; Jama 1993; 270:83

Cause: Decline in androgen production secondary to testicular failure as well as hypothalamic hyporesponsiveness and excessive binding of testosterone in the plasma; morning peak of testosterone much lower in the elderly

Epidem: 29% of men >80 yr have sex 1×/wk; the probability of erectile dysfunction in men >70 = 67% (Arch Sex Behav 1993;22: 545); there may be multiple causes, vascular or neurologic (48%), diabetes (~17%), psychological problems (~9%), drugs (4%), low testosterone (3%)

Pathophys: Atherosclerosis, clot, or vascular surgery lead to decreased arterial supply to penis; venous leakage; trauma to nerves of the penis from lumbar disc disease, rectal surgery, prostatectomy; diabetic neuropathy; alcoholic peripheral neuropathy; drugs eg β-blockers, alcohol, cimetidine, antipsychotics, antidepressants, lithium, sedative hypnotics, hormones

Sx: Erectile dysfunction or lack of interest or decreased mobility; failure to reach ejaculation is very common and can be missed if not asked about

Si: Gynecomastia, diminished male-pattern hair suggests endocrine etiology; abdominal/femoral bruits suggest vascular disease; penile size may prevent effectiveness of suction device; fibrous bands or plaques on penis suggest Peyronie's disease; penile-brachial index after 3–5 min bicycling w legs in air to dx pelvic steal; nocturnal tumescence not reliable; testicular atrophy suggests hypogonadism; absence of vibratory sense or neural reflex arcs suggests neuropathy; review meds; couple discussion helpful

Crs: Intermittent course suggests psychogenic origin while progressive suggests organic; however, chronic illness course may cause intermittency also

Lab: Testosterone level, LH, FBS, urine zinc level, prolactin level, liver function

Xray:

> **Noninvasive:** Nocturnal penile tumescence suggests psychogenic etiology; duplex Doppler US delineates arterial, sinusoidal venous

insufficiency; all usually not necessary and can be gleaned by asking about nighttime erections

Rx:

Therapeutic:
- Avoid drugs w adverse effects of sexual dysfunction: calcium channel blockers and ACE inhibitors have the least effect of the antihypertensive meds; phenothiazines cause retrograde ejaculation; minor tranquilizers affect the limbic system, decreasing libido; MAO inhibitors, tertiary amine tricyclics, cimetidine, digoxin, progestational agents, heparin, estrogen
- Treat hypothyroidism, diabetes
- Mechanical: have spouses of COPD pts assume the superior position in sexual intercourse
- Low testosterone: treat w testosterone im q 2 wk or testosterone patches; replacing testosterone in men increases strength, libido, well-being, osteoporosis (Androderm patch) (Geriatrics 1995;50:52); side effects of therapy: BPH, painful gynecomastia, polycythemia, HT, CHF; Testoderm must be worn on scrotum, less rash than w Androderm (Med Let 1996;38:47); if trial of testosterone fails, check prolactin
- Replace zinc in pts w hyperzincuria: 70 mg elemental zinc/d (J Am Ger Soc 1988;36:57)
- Vascular or neurologic etiology: alprostadil (Nejm 1996;334:873; 1997;336:1); topical prostaglandin E_1 (J Urol 1995;153:1828; Clin Diabetes 1996;14:111); if unsuccessful, try penile prostheses (80% success rate): self contained hydraulic (Flexi-Flate and Hydroflex models) or cable spring (Omnipphase); low satisfaction w intracavernosal prostaglandin injection; angioplasty disappointing results; vacuum erection devices: 70%–90% satisfaction rate
- Discussion of adaptation over time is warranted since many men come to understand that sexuality and sexual intimacy are not dependent on capacity to perform intercourse alone

2. Health Care Maintenance

ARTERIOSCLEROTIC CARDIOVASCULAR DISEASE

BLOOD PRESSURE

Jama 1995; 274:570; U.S. Preventive Services Task Force, Guide to clinical preventive services, Williams & Wilkins, 1989; Ann IM 1988; 108:70; Canadian Task Force on the periodic health examination, Ottawa, Canada Communication Group, 1994

Issues: Systolic Hypertension in Elderly Persons (SHEP) study—systolic HT significantly decreased the incidence of stroke among the young-old (Jama 1991;265:3255; Canadian Task Force 1994:943)
Benefits may not be demonstrable among the old-old (Jama 1994; 272:1932; Lancet 1995;345:825; J Hypertens Suppl 1986;4:S642); mortality inversely related to elevated systolic and diastolic BP in those patients aged 85 and older (BMJ 1988;296:887); however, higher rates of fatal MI in men w pharmacologically induced diastolic BP decrease from 90 to 86 mmHg (J Hypertens 1994;12: 1183); 20% of elderly whose antihypertensive meds withdrawn while normotensive remained normotensive, whereas 80% of those withdrawn from hypertensive therapy required resumption of treatment in 3 mo to 1 yr (J Intern Med 1994;235:581)

Intervention: Screen NH pts for HT, but use caution in treating those >80 yr; periodic trial off meds, particularly if life becomes more sedentary (eg, pts w progressive disabilities, NH pts)

PULSE

Ann IM 1988;108:70; Canadian Task Force on the periodic health examination, Ottawa, Canada Communication Group, 1994

Issues: Risk of stroke for pts w Afib w at least one other risk factor (HT, DM, TIA, h/o stroke) is 8%
Intervention: Check pulse in pts in whom aspirin or warfarin would be considered (Arch IM 1994;154:1443,1449)

PALPATION ABDOMINAL AORTA WIDTH

Ann IM 1988;108:70; Canadian Task Force on the periodic health examination, Ottawa, Canada Communication Group, 1994

Issues: Palpation for abdominal aortic aneurysm 80%–90% sens; elective nonemergent surgery risk for aneurysm >5 cm = 5% as opposed to emergent 50%–70% mortality rate
Intervention: Palpate abdominal aorta in pt in whom surgery would be considered (Prim Care 1995;22:731)

CAROTID AUSCULTATION

Issues: 55% reduction in relative risk results from endarterectomy in asx pts with >70% stenosis (Circ 1995;91:566), >60% (Jama 1995;273:1421); both Canadian Task Force (1994) and European study (Lancet 1995;345:209) do not advocate endarterectomy for asx pts; carotid bruit auscultation has low specif for carotid stenosis
Intervention: Where high-quality surgical services are available, auscultate carotids in high-risk pts <80 yr who are good surgical candidates (American Academy of Family Practice recommendations, Prim Care 1995;22:731)

CHOLESTEROL

Issues: High prevalence of hypercholesterolemia in asx elderly would require further lipid profiles in f/u, putting an enormous burden on the health care system (J Fam Pract 1992;34:320)

Low HDL cholesterol predicts coronary heart disease mortality in older persons (Jama 1995;274:539)

Computer simulation data suggest that treatment of those with established CAD is more cost-effective than primary prevention in the elderly (Ann IM 1995;122:539)

There have been no clinical trials to assess the risk or benefit of cholesterol-lowering meds in the elderly; inverse relationship between high cholesterol level and death from CAD by age 70–80 (Arch IM 1993;153:1065; Jama 1994;272:1335)

Intervention: Pts w >2 cardiac risk factors (Ann IM 1996;124:515), American Heart Association screen everyone into very old age; those pts with a life expectancy <3 yr should not be screened for hypercholesterolemia; lovastatin extremely well tolerated in older cohort (J Am Ger Soc 1997;45:8)

In *NH* setting, pts with decreased cholesterol may be at more risk than those with elevated cholesterol; low cholesterol indicates poor nutritional status and is associated with a high 6-mo mortality rate (J Am Ger Soc 1991;39:455); clinical trial data lacking

ELECTROCARDIOGRAM

Issues: Screening EKGs have low specif and poorly predict future cardiac events; U.S. Public Service Task Force recommends EKGs in pts with 2 or more cardiac risk factors, but does not specifically address the elderly; discovery of silent ischemia on screening EKG could lead to treatment with significant side effects (Ann IM 1989;111:489)

Intervention: Baseline EKG for diagnostic purposes (comparison) for all NH pts and pts in continuity practices

COUNSELING (SMOKING, EXERCISE, ASPIRIN, ESTROGEN)

Issues: Cardiovascular benefits of smoking cessation do not diminish with age (Nejm 1988;319:1365); American College of Physicians, Canadian Task Force, and U.S. Preventive Task Force recommend smoking cessation; difficult to achieve in the *NH* setting where pt's rights to freedom of choice are invoked

Increasing physical activity reduces the incidence of coronary heart disease in female pts as old as 69 (JAMA 1997;277:1287), HT, NIDDM, colon cancer, depression, and anxiety; decreases cholesterol; and may improve cognition and self-image (Ann Rev Pub Hlth 1987;8:253; Nejm 1986;314:605; 1991;325:147; J Am Ger Soc 1990;38:123; Jama 1984;252:544); decreased episodes of CHF in elderly who walked 4 h/wk at 75% of their maximum heart rate (Jama 1994;272:1442)

Estrogen cardioprotective via beneficial effects on lipid profile (American College Physicians Ann IM 1992;117:1016,1038; Nejm 1992; 326:1406; Nurses study–Nejm 1991;325:756; PEPI trial–JAMA 1995;273:199)

Intervention: Strongly encourage even the very old pt to quit smoking unless life expectancy is <2 yr (J Fam Pract 1992;34:320); do not assume pts who have quit have done so forever, continue to counsel (Prim Care 1995;22:697)

Walking programs for appropriately selected ambulatory pts; weight-bearing exercises that avoid flexion of the spine for osteoporotic pts; Tai Chi (J Am Ger Soc 1996;44:489,498); encourage weight training

U.S. Preventive Task Force recommends aspirin for pts >40 yr with at least 2 risks for CAD (1st-degree relative, smoking, HT, DM, h/o stroke or peripheral vascular disease, obesity, low levels of HDL) (J Am Ger Soc 1990;38:817,933); however in the elderly the benefits may not outweigh the risks of aspirin (ie, gi bleeding) (J Am Board Fam Pract 1992;5:127)

Estrogen Replacement: Avoid menstrual bleeding w daily estrogen 0.625 mg and progesterone 2.5 mg; into very old age because not only cardioprotective but beneficial effects on osteoporosis, Alzheimer's as well? (Byyny RL, Speroff L, A clinical guide for the care of older women, Williams & Wilkins, 1996)

HEALTH CARE MAINTENANCE

CANCER

BREAST CANCER

Issues: Breast cancer less aggressive than in premenopausal women; the more poorly differentiated tumors with less organized cells, ie, no hormone receptors, are selected out by aging, resulting in the more differentiated tumors lasting into old age; according to actuarial statistics healthy 80-yr-old women will live 9 more yr, but most NH pts have medical problems that will shorten their life expectancy

    Morbidity: Fungating tumors, metastasis to bone, liver, lung, and 15% to brain; 50% of asx elderly women with breast cancer may have bony metastases (Ger Med Today 1989;8(7):27); local complications develop in nearly half of untreated 85-yr-old women with a breast lump; a demented 85-yr-old woman has a 75% chance of dying before these complications develop (J Am Ger Soc 1995;43:282)

    Tamoxifen has been used in lieu of surgery in the frail elderly pt who develops breast cancer (Br J Surg 1991;78:591)—easily tolerated and may also protect against osteoporosis

    $\geq$ 4 hr/wk exercise decreases risk of breast cancer (Nejm 1997;336:1269)

Intervention: In selected pts where the likelihood of developing morbidity from breast cancer will precede death from other causes, screen for breast cancer into late life w mammogram as well as breast exam (Lancet 1993;341:1973); up to age 85 yr (J Am Ger Soc 1997;45:344), Medicare covers q 2 yr screening mammography

    In the frail NH pt w average life expectancy: limit screening to a breast exam (Ann IM 1995;122:539)—low-risk rx, eg, tamoxifen, easily available for management

COLON CANCER

U.S. Preventive Services Task Force, Guide to clinical preventive services, 2nd ed, Williams & Wilkins, 1996

Issues: Two-thirds of new cases of colon cancer diagnosed each yr are found in people older than 65 yr; time for polyp to become malignant ranges from 5–12 yr (Ann IM 1991;115:807); dx and rx of colorectal cancer is curative or palliative and may improve quality of life, though perioperative mortality does increase with age

Digital rectal exam, fecal occult blood testing, and sigmoidoscopy: 25% decrease in mortality associated with their use (Nejm 1993; 328:1365; Ann IM 1993;118:1); well-designed case-control studies suggest protection remains unchanged for at least 10 yr after rigid sigmoidoscopy (U.S. Preventive Task Force, 1996); simple occult blood testing can lead to serial colonoscopies, expense, and discomfort without necessarily increasing longevity in debilitated elderly; controversial one-time screening with colonoscopy has been suggested for those >60 yr old (National Polyp Study—Am J Gastroenterol 1994;86:197; Nejm 1993;329:1977; Jama 1994;271:1011)

Interventions:

- General population of well elderly: screening with fecal occult blood tests yearly and sigmoidoscopies every 10 yr appropriate
- Studies of colorectal screening targeting the growing NH population are needed to support more specific recommendations

    The Canadian Task Force finds insufficient evidence of benefit to include or exclude colon cancer screening of individuals >40 yr, asx, or with family hx (Canadian Task Force on the periodic health examination, Ottawa, Canada Communication Group, 1994)

- Take advantage of low cost of fecal occult blood screening and use repeat screening as valuable diagnostic tool when clinical suspicion is high

CERVICAL CANCER

Issues: 40% of cervical cancer deaths occur in women >65 yr; 50% of women >65 yr have never had a pap smear, and an additional 25% have not had regular screening; women >65 who have never had pap smear have 2–3× the risk of younger women for having abnormal pap (Am J Obgyn 1991;164:644); women >65 would benefit more than any age group from cancer screening with a 63% improvement in 5-yr mortality (Lancet 1990;335:97)

Canadian recommendations suggest that 2 neg pap smears are sufficient even in women never previously screened who are >65; cervical cancer screening, according to these guidelines, is about one-sixth the cost of mammography screening per yr of life saved

Women who have had any previous abnormal paps should be screened q 2–3 yr late into life (U.S. Preventive Task Force, 1996); w regularly documented neg pap smears, it is safe and cost-effective to stop screening at age 65 (Ann IM 1992;117:529)

Pathophysiology of Cervix with Aging: As a women ages, the transformation zone migrates further into the cervix and is more difficult for the clinician to visualize; estrogen reverses this change; in order to obtain optimally reliable cytology in high-risk elderly women, use intravaginal estrogen for 3 wk prior to pap smear to avoid false-pos smears, because atrophic changes can be read as atypia on pap smear (Culposcopy course, Santa Fe, NM, 3/95)

Mechanical Barriers to Screening: Pelvic examination not only may be uncomfortable but also may lead to pain in severely arthritic, osteoporotic women; consider using "heels together, knees apart" position w assistant providing lateral knee support (rather than standard stirrups) for increased comfort; demented pts may be unable to cooperate with the procedure; therefore may want to examine in left lateral decubitus position; decreased estrogen also makes vaginal introitus stenotic, shortened, narrowed

Natural History of Disease: The natural hx of untreated cervical cancer usually involves local spread, and subsequent ureteral and bowel obstruction causing death; rx options depend on the stage of the disease, progressing from cryosurgery, loop electrocautery excision procedure, and laser, to surgery and radiation

Intervention: Cost-effective schedule of cervical cancer screening can be limited to previously unscreened women, and women w previous abnormal pap smears who can tolerate the pap smear, culposcopy, and the various rx's for dysplasia and cervical cancer

Other Gynecologic Cancers: Routine screening for ovarian cancer not yet proved to reduce morbidity or mortality (Jama 1995;273:491); a careful hx to elicit abnormal bleeding patterns requiring endometrial bx is the initial screening tool for endometrial cancer (J Fam Pract 1992;34:320)

PROSTATE CANCER

Issues: Most common cancer in men; 2nd leading cause of cancer death in men >75 yr, after lung cancer (J Fam Pract 1992;34:320); >99% of men diagnosed with this disease die of other causes (Prog Clin Biol Res 1988;269:87); the American Cancer Society began recommending the PSA test along with digital rectal exam starting at age 50 for men with a life expectancy of at least 10 yr (CA 1993;43:42); PSA may be more sens for aggressive cancers than nonaggressive cancers and may advance detection of early prostate cancer by 5.5 yr (Jama 1995;273:269)

Despite earlier detection of cancer and subsequent prostatectomy in the U.S., there has been no change in the incidence of advanced disease or overall mortality; 1% incidence of death with prostatectomy is about the same as the chance of dying of the prostate cancer itself for an older male (Lancet 1994;343:251); other risks of surgery include impotence and incontinence (often hidden by the pt); benefit of screening offset by morbidity of treatment (Jama 1994;272:773); long-term survival after conservative treatment of localized prostate cancer not changed with low-grade tumors (Jama 1995;274:626)

Interventions: Prostate cancer screening and rx are controversial even in otherwise well men and contraindicated in most NH pts whose average life expectancy is much less than 10 yr; rapidly developing literature demands attention by physicians and discussion w pts before screening

SKIN CANCER

Aging of the skin, in Hazzard WR, Bierman EL, Blass J, et al, eds, The principles of geriatric medicine and gerontology, 3rd ed, McGraw-Hill, 1994:411

Issues: Mortality from melanoma has increased by 50% in women >65 yr and by 100% in men >65 yr; high incidence of actinic keratoses combined w low incidence of conversion to squamous cell carcinoma; even basal cell carcinomas may rapidly disfigure, making early detection important to the pt

Intervention: U.S. Preventive Task Force recommends screening pts w yearly exam with increased sun exposure and with a family hx of dysplastic nevi; important for primary care provider to follow all abnormal lesions w serial exams for cost-effective management

ORAL CANCER

Issues: Tongue cancer most common (~26%), then oropharynx (~22%), then lip (~19%), then floor of the mouth (~16%), then gingiva (~19%), then buccal mucosa (~3%), then hard palate (~2%); speckled leukoplakia, erythroplakia carry more risk than leukoplakia; <50% elderly survive oral cancer; 50% of elderly have undetected gum disease which can have a systemic impact on health; xerostomia common in NH elderly, especially those on anticholinergic drugs (AJN 1995;81:1135)

Intervention: Screen pts with a hx of tobacco or alcohol use for oral cancer, and other problems of the oral cavity as well; although there are no well-designed controlled, cohort studies that prove dental screening effective in the elderly, it is easy to screen yearly with an oral cavity exam (Gerodontics 1988;4:207)

INFECTION CONTROL

INFECTION SURVEILLANCE

Clin Ger Med 1992;8:1821; Yoshikawa TT, Norman DC, eds, Antimicrobial therapy in the elderly patient, 1994; Clin Ger Med 1995;11: 467; Nurs Home Med 1995;3:207

Issues:

Nursing Home: Endemic (UTI, URI, skin), and epidemic (influenza,TB, gastroenteritis); approximately 1 infection/resident/yr; fever criterion should be lowered to 99° (rectal) or 100° (oral), and temperature rise of 2°F from baseline should be viewed as febrile response (J Am Ger Soc 1996;44:74); atypical clinical manifestations: anorexia, falling, incontinence, mental status change; methicillin-resistant *Staphyloccocus aureus* (MRSA) infection: 10%–25% of NH pts colonized, but only 3%–5% infected

Intervention:

Nursing Home: Develop daily reporting system that includes criteria for infection, for nursing staff to use, from which infection rates in the NH can be determined

MRSA-colonized pts do not require isolation, but should not share room w pts w gastric feeding tubes, wounds, iv catheters, or immunosuppression

Vancomycin-resistant enterococci (VRE) (Nurs Home Med 1997;4: 371): contact precautions for colonized or infected pts include grouping pts in same room, wearing gloves and gowns if pt or environmental surface contact anticipated, dedicating frequently used equipment, and barriers for shared equipment, eg, exercise machines; VRE infection control includes surveillance stool cultures or rectal swabs of roommates of newly discovered VRE-colonized pts; may remove contact precautions when 3 neg VRE cultures separated by weekly intervals

TUBERCULOSIS

Issues: Declining immune system leads to reactivation of quiescent infection; chronic cough, weight loss incorrectly attributed to COPD, or malnutrition could result in unrecognized TB epidemic
Intervention:
> **Nursing Home:** Screen new admissions; screen staff yearly; screen pts yearly if high prevalence of TB in community and NH
> • If PPD <10 mm after 48 h, booster in 2 wk
> • Use dermal controls for immunocompromised
> • F/u pos PPD w chest xray and obtain 6 morning sputums for AFB
>
> Chemoprophylaxis: rx conversion of >15 mm within 2 yr with INH 300 mg, pyridoxine 50 mg × 6 mo, check AST q 3 mo, discontinue rx if AST rises to 3 × nl, rechallenge once AST nl, with 50 mg INH, increasing by 50 mg weekly to 300 mg/d; do not rechallenge if AST rises again

DECUBITUS ULCER

Issues: Prevalence in NH >20%–30% incurs fourfold risk of death
Intervention: Norton or Braden scales (see pressure sores, p 248)
> screen for risk of decubiti, taking physical and mental condition, activity level, mobility, and incontinence into account; for pts at high risk: ensure adequate repositioning schedules, check albumin, and order high-protein diets (J Am Diet Assoc 1994;94:1301) (Table 2-1)

Table 2-1. Braden Scale for Predicting Pressure Sore Risk

Patient's Name _____   Evaluator's Name _____   Date of Assessment

	1	2	3	4		
SENSORY PERCEPTION Ability to respond meaningfully to pressure-related discomfort	1. Completely Limited: Unresponsive (does not moan, flinch, or grasp) to painful stimuli, due to diminished level of consciousness or sedation. OR limited ability to feel pain over most of body surface.	2. Very Limited: Responds only to painful stimuli. Cannot communicate discomfort except by moaning or restlessness. OR has a sensory impairment which limits the ability to feel pain or discomfort over 1/2 of body.	3. Slightly Limited: Responds to verbal commands, but cannot always communicate discomfort or need to be turned. OR has some sensory impairment which limits ability to feel pain or discomfort in 1 or 2 extremities.	4. No Impairment: Responds to verbal commands. Has no sensory deficit which would limit ability to feel or voice pain or discomfort.		
MOISTURE Degree to which skin is exposed to moisture	1. Constantly Moist: Skin is kept moist almost constantly by perspiration, urine, etc. Dampness is detected every time patient is moved or turned.	2. Very Moist: Skin is often, but not always moist. Linen must be changed at least once a shift.	3. Occasionally Moist: Skin is occasionally moist, requiring an extra linen change approximately once a day.	4. Rarely Moist: Skin is usually dry, linen only requires changing at routine intervals.		
ACTIVITY Degree of physical activity	1. Bedfast: Confined to bed	2. Chairfast: Ability to walk severely limited or non-existent. Cannot bear own weight and/or must be assisted into chair or wheelchair.	3. Walks Occasionally: Walks occasionally during day, but for very short distances, with or without assistance. Spends majority of each shift in bed or chair.	4. Walks Frequently: Walks outside the room at least twice a day and inside room at least once every 2 hours during waking hours.		
MOBILITY Ability to change and control body position	1. Completely Immobile: Does not make even slight changes in body or extremity position without assistance.	2. Very Limited: Makes occasional slight changes in body or extremity position but unable to make frequent or significant changes independently.	3. Slightly Limited: Makes frequent though slight changes in body or extremity position independently.	4. No Limitations: Makes major and frequent changes in position without assistance.		

NUTRITION *Usual* food intake pattern	1. Very Poor: Never eats a complete meal. Rarely eats more than 1/3 of any food offered. Eats 2 servings or less of protein (meat or dairy products) per day. Takes fluids poorly. Does not take a liquid dietary supplement. OR is NPO and/or maintained on clear liquids or IV's for more than 5 days.	2. Probably Inadequate: Rarely eats a complete meal and generally eats only about 1/2 of any food offered. Protein intake includes only 3 servings of meat or dairy products per day. Occasionally will take a dietary supplement. OR receives less than optimum amount of liquid diet or tube feeding.	3. Adequate: Eats over half of most meals. Eats a total of 4 servings of protein (meat, dairy products) each day. Occasionally will refuse a meal, but will usually take a supplement if offered. OR is on a tube feeding or TPN regimen which probably meets most of nutritional needs.	4. Excellent: Eats most of every meal. Never refuses a meal. Usually eats a total of 4 or more servings of meat and dairy products. Occasionally eats between meals. Does not require supplementation.
FRICTION AND SHEAR	1. Problem: Requires moderate to maximum assistance in moving. Complete lifting without sliding against sheets is impossible. Frequently slides down in bed or chair, requiring frequent repositioning with maximum assistance. Spasticity, contractures or agitation leads to almost constant friction.	2. Potential Problem: Moves feebly or requires minimum assistance. During a move skin probably slides to some extent against sheets, chair, restraints, or other devices. Maintains relatively good position in chair or bed most of the time but occasionally slides down.	3. No Apparent Problem: Moves in bed and in chair independently and has sufficient muscle strength to lift up completely during move. Maintains good position in bed or chair at all times.	

Total Score

For additional information on administration and scoring refer to the following reference:

1. Braden BJ, Bergstrom N. Clinical utility of the Braden Scale for Predicting Pressure Sore Risk. *Decubitus* 1989;2(3):44–51.

IMMUNIZATIONS

INFLUENZA

Issues: 4th leading cause of death pts >75 yr; 70% *NH* residents contact influenza during outbreak, 10%–20% in nonepidemic years; fatality rate 30%; immunization rate 20%–40% because physicians don't communicate and pts don't understand seriousness of illness (Clin Ger Med 1992;8:183); cost-effective saving $117/person, $5 million in cumulative savings (Nejm 1994;331:778)

Intervention: Aim to immunize 80% NH pts (Jama 1994;272:1133); during outbreaks begin prophylaxis regardless of vaccination status to both ill and non-ill pts; rimantadine has fewer CNS side effects, more expensive than amantadine (Geriatrics 1994;49:30); reduce side effects of amantadine by dosing according to calculated creatinine clearance, and decreasing other anticholinergic meds

PNEUMOCOCCAL PNEUMONIA

Issues: Increased incidence by 2–4× in pts >65 yr; 20% vaccination rate, partially due to low Medicaid/Medicare reimbursement through 1989

Intervention: Aim to vaccinate 60% NH pts; revaccinate q 6 yr in elderly w asplenia, nephrotic syndrome, or renal failure; revaccination w 23-valent vaccine should be considered for pts who were vaccinated w 14-valent vaccine (Am Fam Phys 1995;51:859)

TETANUS

Issues: Increased incidence with age because protective antitoxin levels decline; 28% have protective levels over the age of 70 (Nejm 1995;332:761); 10% pts are fecal carriers of *Clostridium tetani*, leaving pressure ulcers at high risk for contamination; case fatality rate = 50%

Intervention: Give tetanus immune globulin to pts with contaminated ulcers who have completed primary series but have not had reimmunization within 10 yr; give primary series to pts with unknown immunization status; pts in the military after 1941 have received at least one tetanus toxoid dose (Inf Contr Hosp Epidem 1993;14: 591)

FUNCTION

FUNCTIONAL ASSESSMENT

Issues: Emphasize quality of life issues over extension of life; screening with this goal in mind emphasizes preservation of function; the Canadian Task Force and the U.S. Preventive Task Force recommend screening for functional assessment in the elderly

INTERVENTION

In Office and NH: Nurses perform a yearly functional assessment (Kane RL, Ouslander JG, Abrass IB, Essentials of clinical geriatrics, 3rd ed, McGraw-Hill, 1993)

Katz functional assessment is one of the most common; assesses actual capacity and not performance, and records loss of independence in 6 skills in the order in which they are lost; bathing, dressing, toileting, transferring, continence, and feeding; they are usually regained in the reverse order

SENSORY—HEARING AND VISION

HEARING

Issues: The Canadian Task Force and U.S. Preventive Task Force recommend screening for hearing loss in the elderly; particularly effective screen in the old-old pt (J Fam Pract 1992;34:320); 41% of pts >65 yr are hearing impaired (Ear Hear 1990;11:247)

Intervention: Whispered voice, and otoscopy most sens and specif screens (86%–96%) (Ann IM 1990;113:138; Canadian Task Force, 1994); observation of listening behavior helpful; obtain a hx of hearing loss, perform otoscopy for cerumen impaction, and f/u w portable audiometry for presbycusis where indicated; pts sometimes refuse to wear hearing aids; ascertain the cause of their noncompliance, eg, poorly fit, difficult to manipulate, change in hearing deficit, depression, dementia, rather than assuming indifference or stubbornness

VISION

Issues:

Community: 9% >65 yr, 50% >75 yr have visual impairment, optical changes in aging (Mangione CM, Intensive Course in Geriatric Medicine and Board Review, 1/96)

- Increased light absorption by crystalline lens reducing intensity reaching photoreceptors
- Senile miosis: older pupils smaller, leading to less light getting to retina in low-light conditions
- Increased intraocular light scatter, leading to heightened sensitivity to glare
- Decreased amplitude of accommodation of the lens (presbyopia) so by 60 or 70 yr most need glasses for near vision
- Axis of astigmatism changes, requiring refraction
- Neural change w loss of blue-yellow discrimination; no prospective studies to show that screening the elderly for visual acuity is worthwhile, however

Nursing Home: 17% of pts in NHs blind and another 19% have <20/40 vision; 20% of blindness and 37% of impairment remediable with adequate refraction (Nejm 1995;332:1205); Baltimore eye study: unoperated cataracts accounted for 27% of all blindness in blacks, suggesting that elderly with less access to eye care would benefit from screening for cataracts (Nejm 1991;325: 1412; Mangione CM, 1996)

Macular degeneration leading cause of blindness among whites (3% of all whites >80 yr); early treatment w laser effective in slowing progression; referral to low vision services may help pt to maximize peripheral vision

Diabetic retinopathy most treatable in presymptomatic phase when neovascular changes have just begun

Impaired visual acuity linked to falls and hip fractures; therefore screening the old-old may be beneficial (Nejm 1991;324:1326)

Screen using combination of visual field exam, tonometry, and direct ophthalmoscopy by ophthalmologist w pt's eyes completely dilated (2.5% phenylephrine w tear duct occlusion to decrease systemic absorption), long asx and potentially treatable phase before irreversible vision loss (UCLA intensive board review, 1/96). However, reliable screening tests for glaucoma are not available and early treatment does not improve pt outcome (Surv Ophthalmol 1983;28:194)

Intervention: Screen for visual acuity yearly; visual acuity screening criteria for referral to specialist: best eye <20/40 (wearing correction), >2 Snellen lines difference between two eyes; hx of night driving problems helpful for accident prevention

MENTAL HEALTH ISSUES

DEMENTIA

Nejm 1990;322:1212

Issues: Screening recommended by the American College of Physicians, Canadian Task Force, and U.S. Preventive Task Force; Mini Mental State Exam (MMSE) has a broad range; moderate but not mild deficits can be picked up; Wechsler identifies subtle deficit, but lengthy to administer; 4–7-yr delay in presentation to health care provider

Intervention: Use MMSE (Folstein, Bar Harbor, ME, 6/96) to pick up attention span deficit associated with the reversible dementias (and delirium), ie, thyroid disorders, other metabolic abnormalities, and acute infections; MMSE helps identify the type and stage of dementia; prevent unnecessary agitation in demented pts by providing stage-appropriate challenges without overstimulating them with activities that are too difficult for them; careful spouse and family hx probably undervalued as dx tool

DEPRESSION

Issues: 10%–15% of general geriatric population depressed; 60% of NH elderly may be depressed; masked depression more common among the elderly presenting w agitation, jealousy, or somatization

Intervention: Asking single question "Have you been feeling depressed?" may be just as effective as Geriatric Depression Scale (GDS) (J Am Ger Soc 1994;42:1006); anhedonia (failure to find usual pleasures) can be sensitive sx; GDS only requires yes/no answers, has a shortened form, but may lack specif among medically ill pts; Beck, Zung, and Hamilton depression inventories rely heavily on somatic complaints and therefore are less useful in the elderly; nonverbal depression scale developed by Hayes and Losche is useful in more debilitated NH pts (Clin Gerontol 1991;10:3)

ALCOHOL PROBLEMS

J Am Ger Soc 1995;43:415

Issues: Prevalence of alcohol problems = 10% in community; in the *NH* ranges from 2.8%–15%; one-third of the pts who enter a NH will return to their community, thereby making alcohol rehabilitation more relevant (Ger Rev Syllabus 1996). Knowledge of ETOH hx may add to the understanding of family-pt interactions, behaviors exhibited with the staff such as "dry drunk" spells will take on new meaning as well; move to retirement communities associated w increased ETOH use

Intervention: Screening with either a CAGE or MAST-G yields 82%/ 90% and 93%/65% sens/specif rates, respectively (Ger Rev Syllabus 1996); CAGE not reliable as only screening tool in outpatients >60 yr; clinicians should directly ask about number of drinks per week (Jama 1996;276:1964); watch for reluctance to appropriately modify ETOH use w illness, new meds; pointing out percentage of daily calories provided by 1, 2, 3, etc. drinks, may help to improve nutrition

Issues:

Community: Lower extremity dysfunction predicts subsequent disability (Nejm 1995;332:556); one-leg balance important indicator of injurious falls (J Am Ger Soc 1997;45:735); slowed timed chair stands, decreased arm strength, decreased vision and hearing, high anxiety or depression score also predictors for falls (Jama 1995;273:1348)

Nursing Home: Increased fall rates in NH residents after relocation in a new facility (J Am Ger Soc 1995;43:1237); pts who fall infrequently are at most risk for injury; they tend to be going at faster speeds at point of impact; these pts as well as those who fall frequently can be helped by an intervention which determines the etiology of their falls; fear of falling leads to functional decline (Gerontol 1994;40:38), and should be considered important part of all fall management

Interventions: (See pp 206–208, osteoporosis, hip fracture) Screen all outpatients and ambulatory NH pts with an assessment of balance and gait; Tinetti assessment tool (J Am Ger Soc 1986;34:119) evaluates normal, and adaptive, ability to maintain balance when arising from a chair, standing with eyes closed, turning, and receiving a sternal nudge; also evaluates several components of gait (step height, postural sway, path deviation); abnormalities in particular parts of the exam point to specific intrinsic etiologies of falling, eg, "uses arms to assist in standing—may have proximal muscle weakness and might be helped by strength training for hip and quad muscles"; foot scuff during swing phase—anterior tibial muscle weakness which might be aided by an ankle/foot orthosis or reconditioning; observational gait analysis (see p 57)

Prevent falls by using both intrinsic and extrinsic approaches; increased muscle strength is associated with decreased falling (J Am Ger Soc 1994;42:953); exercise training decreases falls (Jama 1995;273:1341); work with physical therapist to develop a care plan; use antigravity exercises that do not flex the spine, to avoid vertebral compression fractures in severely osteoporotic pts

Osteoporosis likely in pts whose height has decreased on yearly screening; high risk: white, Asian, thin, nulliparous, sedentary, kyphotic women with past or family hx of fracture, both men and women who smoke, have COPD, or take steroids chronically; postmenopausal estrogen therapy at any age prevents further bone loss and serious injury from falls; if no preexisting breast cancer, prescribe estrogen (several different regimens see p 15), vs estrogen begun 5 yr after menopause no fracture prevention benefit at any site (Ann IM 1995;122:9); calcitonin via intranasal route is an option for pts with fracture pain in whom estrogen is contraindicated, but costly (Ann IM 1992,117:1038); alendronate (see osteoporosis, p 208)

Hip fractures reduced by 23% when adequate calcium supplementation prescribed (1.2 gm/d) with 800 IU of vit D (Osteoporos Int 1994;4(suppl 1):7); adequate levels of vit D found in most OTC vit supplements (J Endocrinol Metab 1995;80:1052); unless elderly women have a hx of renal stones, should have total calcium intake = 1.2 gm/d and add vit D if they are not exposed to direct sunlight for at least one-half hour a day; a serving of broccoli or dairy product equivalent to 1 Tums tab, which is 0.2 gm of elemental calcium; use this as a guide to decide calcium tab supplementation

Extrinsic approaches: hip pads and chariot ambulators maintain independent walking, prevent serious injury (Lancet 1993;341:11); restraint reduction not increase serious falls (J Am Ger Soc 1994; 42:321,960; Arch IM 1992;116:368); evaluate meds: sedatives, narcotics, neuroleptics, and antihypertensives (Table 2-2).

INCONTINENCE

Urinary Incontinence Guideline Panel, Urinary incontinence in adults: clinical practice guideline, AHCPR Publc No. 92-0038, Rockville, MD, Agency for Health Care Policy and Research, Public Health Service, U.S. Dept. of Health and Human Services, 3/92

Issues: 50% of NH pts incontinent of urine resulting in social embarrassment and medical complications such as skin infections; high hidden prevalence in both men and women in community

Interventions: (See p 30) Screen for reversible causes of incontinence, ie, local causes: bladder infection, atrophic vaginitis, stool impaction; functional causes: delirium, depression, immobility; systemic ill-

Table 2-2. Observational Gait Analysis

3 × 3 × 3 MODEL

Ask: Which of the three essential components is involved?

1. **FOOT CLEARANCE IN SWING**
2. **UPRIGHT SUPPORT IN STANCE**
3. **CONTROLLED FORWARD MOVEMENT**

Then Ask: Where does the problem occur?

1. **GATHERING INFORMATION**
2. **PROCESSING INFORMATION**
3. **PRODUCING MOVEMENT**

Finally: What can be done?

1. **PREVENTION**
2. **CORRECTION**
3. **COMPENSATION**

FOOT CLEARANCE IN SWING PHASE	UPRIGHT SUPPORT IN STANCE PHASE	CONTROLLED FORWARD MOVEMENT
	Gathering Information	
Proprioceptive loss *Compensatory strategy: orthotics hard-soled shoes*	Paresthesias *Preventative strategy: foot care*	Vestibular disturbance *Corrective strategy: desensitization exercises*
	Processing Information	
Poor coordination	Polypharmacy	Difficulty initiating or terminating movement, e.g., Parkinson's disease
Compensatory strategy: enhance safety with architectural redesign	*Corrective strategy: streamline medication*	*Preventative strategy: prevent secondary problems of weakness, inflexibility, and poor joint mobility*
	Movement Production	
Tight gastroc-soleus, eg, 15° of ankle dorsiflexion necessary for normal gait	Weak hip abductors, eg, Trendelenburg	Arthritis pain
Corrective strategy: stretching	*Corrective strategy: strengthening*	*Preventative strategy: shock-absorbing inserts, prevent deconditioning*

Data from C Rosemond, PT, GCS, University of North Carolina, Chapel Hill.

nesses: CHF, hyperglycemia; meds: anticholinergic, and α-adrenergic agents; diet: excess caffeine, soda, alcohol ("bladder irritants")

Collaborate with nurses to determine the etiology of incontinence, obtaining significant positive hx for urge, stress, overflow, or functional incontinence; fluid intake, voiding pattern, PVR volume, and UA complete the w/u necessary for empiric rx; screening in this way will allow for identification of a select number of pts who are likely to respond to bladder retraining, an intervention requiring significant staff time and commitment; careful management of early dx and management (change of habits, exercise, meds) of community elderly can be rewarding

SEXUAL FUNCTION

Nurs Home Med 1995;3:56

Issues: 70% of male NH residents and 50% of female NH residents have thought about being close or intimate (Arch Sex Behav 1988;17:109); sexual contacts often casual and involve manual or oral genital stimulation, rather then coitus; privacy rooms often lacking or ill equipped for a couple engaging in a mutual sexual act, even for an able-bodied couple; private space infrequently made for heterosexually wedded couples, almost never made available for gay, lesbian, or bisexual couples; public masturbation may occur when pts seek out stairwells or alcoves, attempting to be out of the scrutiny of the staff

67% of men >80 yr have sex 1×/wk; primary reason older women do not have sex is unavailability of partner (Arch Sex Behav 1993; 22:543; 1994;23:231) (also see pp 36–37)

Intervention: Remove barriers to sexual expression by encouraging privacy (do-not-disturb signs, closed doors), allowing conjugal or home visits, evaluating complaints of sexual function, and changing meds that may affect sexual function; council interested pts about sexuality, assess decision making capacity of impaired elderly, and provide staff education (Am Fam Phys 1995;51:121)

Outpatient: Educational counseling to increase pt's comfort in addressing sexual issues and enlarge views of sexuality to link w larger intimacy issues and wide variation a "healthy" sexual adaptation

OTHER ANTICIPATORY MEASURES

ADVANCED DIRECTIVES

Ouslander JG, Osterweil D, Morley J, Ethical and legal issues, in Medical care in the nursing home, McGraw-Hill, 1991:358

Issues: Definition of medical futility nebulous; pts >69 have a 5% chance of surviving CPR, but physicians underestimate what pts consider futile; some pts would consider these odds encouraging, and preferable to death (Jama 1995;273:156; Ann IM 1989;111:199); demented pts may be capable of making *some* decisions about their health care (Jama 1995;273:124; 1988;260:797), eg, options regarding a gangrenous leg may be more difficult to comprehend than whether or not to do CPR (J Am Board Fam Pract 1992;5:127)

Pts and families may fear that advanced directives are not readily carried out in many hospitals; failure of pts to review advanced directives w adult children may lead to conflicts within the family at the time of health crisis; strength of documents can depend on regular reiterations of values and wishes to personal physician recorded in medical record

Intervention: End-of-life decisions should be discussed with the pt or their guardian and family members if agreeable in the case of incapacity; include discussion of the following: CPR, ventilator support, hospital or ICU admission, blood transfusion, iv therapy, tube feeding, antibiotics; values questionnaires may be useful to help facilitate discussions (Arch Fam Med 1994;3:1057); early discussions (time of dx of terminal illnesses, including dementia) helpful

MEDICATIONS

Nurs Home Med 1995;3:6

Issues: Risk of adverse drug reaction directly proportional to number of meds pt is on (Ger Rev Syllabus, 1996, Book 1, 3rd ed., p 31); The Omnibus Budget Reconciliation Act of 1987 (OBRA) mandates strict review of psychotropic meds; psychotropic usage has decreased by 50% since OBRA implementation; use same principles for nonpsychiatric drugs

Table 2-3. Lab Work to Follow Effects of Medications for NH Patients

Practice	Frequency
Pts on NSAIDs: check BUN, cr, hct	q 2 mo
Pts on iron replacement: hct	q mo until stable, then q 3 mo
Pts on diuretics: BUN, cr	q 4 mo
Pts on digoxin, phenytoin, quinidine, procaine amide, theophylline, nortriptyline	Levels q 6 mo
cbc, FBS, lytes, BUN, albumin	Yearly
EKG	On admission

Modified from Ann IM 1994;121:584.

Intervention:

> **Community:** If pt has multiple physicians, use "brown bag" strategy to determine complete med list (Prim Care 1995;22:697)
>
> **Nursing Home:** Avoid excessive dosing frequency, prolonged duration of med, duplicate therapy, and side effects that outweigh the benefits of the drug; do not add a med to relieve the side effects of another medicine except perhaps when using anticholinergics to treat extrapyramidal side effects, progesterone to oppose estrogen replacement, or misoprostol to prevent NSAID gastritis; consider cost; interdisciplinary teams including consultant pharmacists can review drug-drug and disease-drug interactions regularly; consider all drugs candidates for regular re-evaluation (Table 2-3)

ELDER ABUSE

Prim Care 1993;20:375; Nejm 1995;332:437; J Am Ger Soc 1994;42: 169; 1996;44:65

Issues: Prevalence not well documented; family, caregivers, and other neighbors of community-dwelling elderly, other NH residents, NH staff, or visitors may be implicated in acts of abuse; stressed caregiver, when worn out by pts w significant functional disabilities represent the overwhelming majority (Canadian Task Force, 1994)

> **Nursing Home:** Inadequate and inconsistent training of caregivers

may contribute to abuse; in one study 10% of nursing assistants admitted to at least one act of physical abuse and 40% admitted to at least one act of psychological abuse in the preceding year

Poor hygiene, signs of dehydration, multiple skin lesions with various degrees of healing, wrist or ankle restraint bruises, and pain with occult fractures; may be subtle: unjustified chemical restraint, verbal and emotional attack, or failure to follow an appropriate care plan; pts with cognitive and physical impairment, and violent, disruptive, or annoying behavior are at particular risk for abuse.

Assess environment early

Baseline physical exam and long-term perspective may allow the physician to perceive changes in demeanor such as withdrawal, depression, or injuries that suggest abuse

Question capable residents directly to clarify any concerns of abuse or neglect: Has anyone ever tried to hurt you? Has anyone ever made you do things you didn't want to do? Has anyone ever taken anything away from you without your consent?

Evaluate mental status to validate the hx, check driving status

Address spiritual concerns

Interview family members, close friends, and staff to determine general social, psychological status and support; differences in details of unlikely explanations of events from various parties may heighten suspicions of abuse; document physical abuse with photographs where possible (Public Health Service, U.S. Dept. of Health and Human Services, AHCPR Publc No. 92-0038, 3/92)

In most states it is mandatory to report suspected abuse to the ombudsmen (U.S. Preventive Services Task Force, Guide to clinical preventive services: an assessment of the effectiveness of 169 interventions, Williams & Wilkins, 1996)

Intervention:

Community: Home care agencies, volunteer organizations, adult daycare, other forms of respite

Nursing Home: Weekly decompression groups for staff to discuss their feelings of frustration in caring for challenging pts provide a forum for creative and constructive changes in care plans; behavioral modification techniques

3. Endocrinology

DIABETES MELLITUS

Am Fam Phys monograph 1995;1:1; Sci Am Med 1995;9:VI; Ger Rev
Syllabus 1996, p. 298

Cause: Resistance to effects of insulin peripherally as well as impaired
insulin release w aging (Diabetes 1991;40:44); secondary causes:
glucocorticoids, hydrochlorothiazide, β-blockers, estrogen, hemochromatosis, Cushing's, acromegaly, pheochromocytoma

Epidem: Frank diabetes in 10% patients >65 yr, 20%–40% of patients
>80 yr old; half the cases of NIDDM not diagnosed (Diabetes
Care 1993;16:642); 18% prevalence, Mexican Americans—3×
risk in whites and 3× risk in whites of severe retinopathy (Diabetes 1988;37:878); native Americans—5× risk in whites (Diabetes
1987;36:523); end-stage renal disease 4.3× higher in blacks and
6× higher in Mexican Americans (Nejm 1989;321:1074); associated w 5–10-yr loss of life (Rationale for the management of
non-insulin-dependent diabetes, Cambridge University Press, 1995:
450)

Pathophys: Glucotoxicity leads to both insulin resistance and decreased
insulin production (Diabetes 1985;34:222); genetic peripheral insulin resistance in the obese pt, and increased levels cause eventual
β-cell exhaustion (Ann IM 1990;113:9050); impaired/delayed insulin release response to glucose load also allows hepatic neogenesis
to persist 1–2 h, then insulin overshoot occurs (Nejm 1992;326:
22); more commonly elderly w NIDDM at risk for hyperglycemic
hyperosmolar nonketotic coma (HHNC), secondary to stress, steroids, tube feeding; failure to replace water because of impaired
thirst and mental status increases osmolarity

Sx: Usually atypical presentation, eg, slowly resolving infection, weight
loss, fatigue, weakness, acute confusional states, depression

Si: Necrobiosis lipoidica (95%) = pigmented skin plaques with white lipid center, irregular, atrophic; fatty hepatomegaly; retinopathy w hard exudates, microaneurysms and hemorrhages (photos in Nejm 1993;329:320); neuropathy w decreased sensation, vibratory sense, position sense

Crs: Years before onset of type II diabetes, pts have hypertriglyceridemia, low HDL, and HT; factors affecting diabetes control in the elderly: decreased vision, altered taste, poor dentition, arthritis, tremor; living alone impairs food preparation and consumption, as well as med administration

Cmplc:

- HHNC: hyperglycemia >600 mg/dL without ketosis or ketoacidosis, w severe volume depletion 25% body weight; serum osmolality > 350 mOsm/kg usually compounding an illness; steroid therapy or tube feeding w concentrated carbohydrate solutions

- Cardiovascular disease 2–3× greater in type II DM than general population; MI and peripheral vascular disease cause 60% of deaths from type II DM, half of nontraumatic amputations due to type II DM (Lebovitz HE, ed, Therapy for diabetes mellitus and related disorders, 2nd ed, American Diabetes Association, 1994)

- Retinopathy: after 15-yr duration, proliferative in 25% of NIDDM on insulin and 5% of those on diet and oral agents (Diabetes Metab Rev 1989;5:559); nonproliferative most common; loss of supporting cells of the retina vasculature leads to microaneurysms, especially at the macula, affecting central vision and visual acuity; when microaneurysms leak, they form punctate "dot-and blot" hemorrhages that then form hard exudates which can cause macular edema if they accumulate near the macula

  With progression of retinopathy, terminal capillaries become obstructed and the retina becomes ischemic; infarctions of the nerve layer cause soft "cotton-wool" exudates; new vessels proliferate in response to ischemia; these new vessels can bleed into the vitreous, which can lead to scars that can retract the retina, leading to retinal detachment and permanent loss of vision

  Type II diabetics also prone to glaucoma, cataracts, corneal abrasions, recurrent corneal erosions, presbyopia

- Nephropathy: highest mortality of all the complications; <20% of pts w NIDDM develop nephropathy (Arch IM 1989;111:788);

begins w microalbuminuria 30–300 mg/24 h; risk factors for nephropathy include duration of DM and HT (Nejm 1988;318:140); inherited tendencies toward ASHD (Nejm 1992;326:673) and w higher infection rates

- Neuropathy: symmetric sensorimotor peripheral neuropathy most common—"stocking-glove"; dysesthesias progress to more severe anesthesia, and neuropathic foot ulcers

  Asymmetric mononeuropathies affecting both peripheral and cranial nerves secondary to nerve infarcts

  Entrapment syndromes such as carpal tunnel syndrome

  Autonomic neuropathy leading to gastroparesis (delayed gastric emptying, early satiety, fullness, nausea, and vomiting), postural hypotension, atonic bladder; polyneuropathy more common in pts w NIDDM and hypoinsulinemia (Nejm 1995;333:89)

  Decreased visceral pain perception, eg, silent angina and MIs (Ann IM 1988;108:170), vs silent MIs not any more common in diabetics (Circ 1996;93:2097)

Lab:

- American Diabetic Association (ADA) criteria: 2 FBS >140 mg/dL, or any random >200; $HbA_{1C} > 7.0$
- Screen w serum fructosamine, marker for short-term diabetic control (J Am Ger Soc 1993;41:1090)
- Monitor HbA_{1C} q 3–6 mo, keep under 8% to avoid microvascular complications; HbA_{1C} increased by Fe deficiency, decreased by sickle cell disease
- Na^+ decreased by increased glucose if not dehydrated; osmoles = 2 $\times$ Na + glucose/18; hence blood sugar/40 $\approx$ 1 Na equivalent

Rx:

Preventive: Annual exams to detect early retinopathy; foot care; detect neuropathy early, screen for microalbuminuria; w tight control of blood sugars there is less progression (J Am Ger Soc 1994;42:142)

Therapeutic:

- For the 85% of diabetics who are obese: low-fat, low-cholesterol diet has highest risk-benefit ratio; aim for fasting cholesterol <200 mg/dL, fasting LDL <130 mg/dL, and <100 if patient has known cardiac disease (Diabetes Care 1993;16:106); fasting triglycerides <200 mg/dL (American Diabetic Association, 1990)
- Weight loss of 5–10 pounds is adequate (BMJ 1975;3:276); dia-

Table 3-1. Oral Hypoglycemic Agents

Drug		Dose Range	Duration of Action
1st gen:	Tolbutamide	500–3000 mg	6–12 h, safest w renal failure
	Tolazamide	100–1000 mg	12–24 h
2nd gen:	Glyburide	2.5–20.0 mg	18–24 h
	Glipizide	5–40 mg	12–18 h

betic pts have more difficulty losing weight than those without; 20% of pts initially control their diabetes by diet alone (Diabetes 1995;44:1249)

- 20-min exercise 3×/wk decreases risk type II diabetes (Nejm 1991;325:147); exercise 1×/wk decreases risk developing DM by 40%, 60% for overweight men
- Stop hyperglycemic-producing meds, eg, estrogen, thiazides, glucocorticoids, sympathomimetics (list—Ann IM 1993; 118:536)
- Conditions requiring drug therapy: sx secondary to hyperglycemia not controlled by diet alone, hyperglycemia leading to risk of dehydration, ketones are present; weight loss is rapid and uncontrolled; hyperlipidemia-hypertriglyceridemia; in elderly, main goal to prevent sx of hyperglycemia, these sx usually begin to occur at glucose concentrations 200–250 mg/dL (Nejm 1996; 334:574)
- Hypoglycemic meds: stimulate endogenous insulin; 2nd-generation hypoglycemics have fewer interactions with other meds than the 1st generations but more frequently cause hypoglycemia, especially the longer acting ones; glyburide more hypoglycemia than glipizide (J Am Ger Soc 1996;44:751); therefore start w low doses and increase every 4–7 d; sustained-release glipizide qd; 20% primary failures and 10%–15% (Table 3-1)
- Insulin has more beneficial effect on lipids (Ann IM 1988;108: 134); tight control, eg, avg HbA_{1C} ≈ (7% w tid insulin prevents neuropathy (Ann IM 1995;122:561—however, no elderly in study); HbA_{1C} <8.1% prevents renal failure (Nejm 1995;332: 1267); hypoglycemia from insulin less prolonged than with oral agents
- Types of insulin: regular—onset 15 min, peak at 4–6 h, duration 6–8 h; NPH—onset in 3 h, peak at 8–12 h, duration 18–24 h;

ENDOCRINOLOGY

Table 3-2. Blood Sugar Management Guidelines

FBS (mg/dL)	Intervention (Sequentially)
126–180	1. Diet
	2. Metformin if overweight, + acarbose if HbA$_{1c}$ 7.5–8.5, and pt tolerates gi adverse effects
	3. Sulfonylureas if lean, + acarbose if HbA$_{1c}$ 7.5–8.5
180–270	1. Sulfonylurea + metformin
	2. Sulfonylurea + 10 pm to 11 pm insulin (Diabetes Med 1992;9:826)
>270	1. Multiple insulin injections (J Fam Pract 1993;36:329)

first-choice regimen (Med Let Drugs Ther 1989;31:363): hs NPH and regular plus NPH in morning; or hs NPH and regular before each meal (Nejm 1993;329:977); start at 5–10 units and increase by 2–3 units every 3–4 d; once stabilized only need to monitor 2 fasting and 2 bedtime measurements a week

- Insulin + oral hypoglycemic: need only 5%–20% of insulin dose required if insulin used alone (Ann IM 1991;115:45)
- Metformin (Biguanide, Glucophage) inhibits gluconeogenesis and induces weight loss (Nejm 1995;333:550); 500–850 mg po hs or bid; increase by 500 mg q 1–2 wk not exceeding 2500 mg; give w meals; won't cause hypoglycemia; give after failure of diet therapy or after sulfonylurea fails; side effects: gi (diarrhea, nausea, anorexia, abdominal discomfort, metallic taste, decreased absorption of vit B$_{12}$, folate); lactic acidosis, especially w liver and renal impairment (abnormal LFTs, Cr >1.5); cardiac or respiratory problems that would lead to hypoxia; severe infection; alcohol abuse; radiographic contrast agents (Nejm 1996;334:577); $47.00/mo (Med Let Drugs Ther 1995;37:41)
- Acarbose: decreases digestion and absorption of disaccharides 25–100 mg po ac tid (Ann IM 1994;121:928); gi side effects may be troublesome (diarrhea, abdominal pain, flatulence); may not want to use w metformin because of additive effects; treat hypoglycemia w glucose not sucrose because sucrose may not be adequately hydrolyzed or absorbed (Med Let Drugs Ther 1996; 38:9) (Table 3-2)
- Troglitazore, a thiazolidinedione, improves insulin resistance without stimulating insulin secretion; give when HbA$_1$c > 8.5% despite insulin rxw > 30 u/d in multiple injections; may also help w HTN, dyslipidemia, atherosclerosis (Clin Diabetes 1997;

15:60); approved by FDA only for use w insulin (200–400 mg gD); cholestyramine absorption (Med Let 1997;39:49)

- Metabolic control of diabetes decreased risk of CHD (Diabetes 1994;43:960), but associated with more driving accidents (J Am Ger Soc 1994;42:695)

- HHNC: look for precipitating infections; replete volume deficit w one-half normal saline; low-dose insulin infusion, 50% mortality; usually don't require insulin rx long term if recover

- Retinopathy: proliferative retinopathy and macular edema respond to laser rx (Ophthalm 1991;98:766); vitrectomy for vitreous scarring may restore sight (Arch Ophthalm 1985;103:1644) (Figure 3-1)

- Nephropathy: control HT, PO_4 restriction (Nejm 1991;324:78), low-protein diets (BMJ 1987;294:295), intensive diabetes rx (Nejm 1993;3329:977), ACE inhibitors prevent proteinuria (Nejm 1993;329:1456; Jama 1994;271:275; Med Let Drugs Ther 1994;36:46; Arch IM 1994;154:625); end-stage renal disease: peritoneal rather than hemodialysis because increased risk of cardiovascular event, and retinal bleed w BP fluctuations and anticoagulation; if renal failure occurs in the absence of proteinuria or retinopathy, search for other etiologies, eg, NSAIDs or UTI

- Neuropathy: rx peripheral neuropathy w tricyclic antidepressants, paroxetine plus imipramine may be more effective than a placebo (Pain 1990;42:135); phenytoin, carbamazepine, capsaicin (which depletes substance P, a pain modulating neurotransmitter, from type C nociceptive fibers) (Arch IM 1991;151:2225)—questionable benefit, $27.00/oz (Med Let Drugs Ther 1992;34.61), rx gastroparesis w metoclopramide, diarrhea w clonidine (Ann IM 1985;102:97) or cisapride (Propulsid); rx impotence w penile vasodilator injections, implantable prostheses, vacuum devices (J Urol 1987;137:678), or prostaglandin injections (Caverjet)—all after appropriate sexual counseling

Team Management:
- Occupational therapy: magnifiers to wrap around syringes, spring filling devices that click, "talking glucometers"; family or nurse may need to do supply setup weekly

- Foot ulcers/infections (Table 3-3) (Nejm 1994;331:854) w anaerobes and *Pseudomonas;* rx w parenteral imipenem or clavulanate potassium–ticarcillin disodium (Timentin) (Sears S, 1991), or

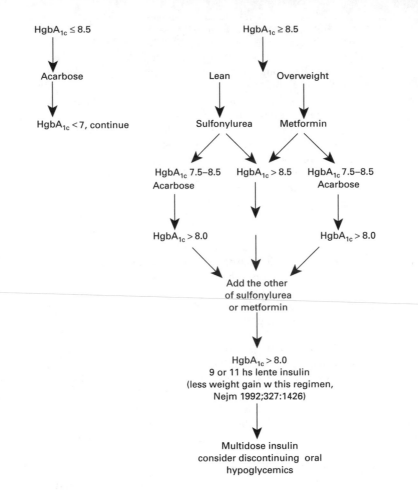

Figure 3-1. Suggested algorithm for type II DM. (Reproduced from Bohamon N, Geriatrics 1996;51:35.)

Table 3-3. Antibiotics in Diabetes

Non-limb-threatening infection

Oral: Cephalexin (Keflex), clindamycin, dicloxacillin, amoxicillin clavulanate (Augmentin)
Parenteral: cefazolin (Ancef), oxacillin, nafcillin, clindamycin

Limb-threatening infection

Oral: fluoroquinolone and clindamycin
Parenteral: same or ampicillin-sulbactam (Unasyn), clavulanate-ticarcillin (Timentin), cefoxitin (Mefoxin), cefotetan (Cefotan)

Life-threatening infection

Imipenem-cilastatin (Primaxin), vancomycin, ampicillin-sulbactam (Unasyn) and aminoglycoside

From Am Fam Phys 1996;53:608.

oral fluoroquinolone plus clindamycin po × 10–14 d; r/o osteomyelitis (Jama 1995;273:712); avoid barefoot walking, get good shoes, rx calluses, check water temperature when bathing feet, toenails clipped straight across

- Medicare coverage for routine foot care (Nurs Home Med 1995; 3:184): one class A finding, or two class B findings, or one class B and two class C findings:

  Class A findings: amputation of foot or integral skeletal portion
  Class B findings: absent posterior tibial pulse, absent dorsalis pedis pulse, 3 advanced trophic changes—decreased hair growth, thickened nails, discoloration, thin skin, rubor
  Class C findings: claudication, cold feet, edema, paresthesia, burning

THYROID

HYPOTHYROIDISM

Clin Ger Med 1995;11:231,239; Jama 1995;273:808; J Am Ger Soc 1993;41:1361; 1994;42:984; 1995;43:592

Cause: Autoimmune thyroiditis; iodine containing drugs decrease thyroid hormone secretion (Nejm 1995;333:1688), eg, radiographic contrast agents; amiodarone (Br J Clin Practice 1993;47:123); cough medicines, eg, codeine phosphate–dextromethorphan hydrobromide (Tussi-Organidin); antiseptic solutions, eg, povidone-iodine (Betadine); long-term lithium (South Med J 1993;86:1182); cholestyramine; aluminum hydroxide; sucralfate (Carafate) decreases T_4 absorption; rarely tumors of pituitary, hypothalamus

Epidem: 2%–5% prevalence; F/M = 5:1; 14% subclinical; risk factors for thyroid failure: family hx of any thyroid disease, hx of hyperthyroidism, subacute thyroiditis, postpartum thyroid disease, radiation (head, neck, chest); other autoimmune disease, eg, Addison's, pernicious anemia; 50% pts with PMR developed hypothyroidism (BMJ 1989;298:647)

Sx: Neither pt nor family aware of changes over number of years; debilitation and apathy (66%); falls (17%); frequently, no, or very few sx

Si:

- Skin: myxedematous infiltration of dermis loosening interface dermal-epidermal layers causing shiny tissue paper appearance; hair loss in scalp
- Head/neck: goiter rare, hoarse voice (0.8%), hypothyroid facies (3.3%) (J Am Ger Soc 1995;43:59); ophthalmologic—primary open-angle glaucoma (Ophthalm 1993;100:1580; Can J Ophthalm 1992;27:341)
- Neurologic: decreased hearing, carpal tunnel syndrome, paresthesias, positional vertigo, myopathy (1.7%)
- Mental status: withdrawn, confused (3.3%), psychotic (Int J Psychiatr Med 1990;20:193), cognitive deficit (J Am Ger Soc 1992:40:325), treatable dementia (Am J Phys Med Rehab 1992;71:28)
- Cardiovascular: effusions (11%), angina (8%), CHF (5.2%), pleural CVA (3.3%), CPK-MB elevated, bradycardia, infrequent HT
- Respiratory: airway obstruction secondary to swollen tongue, pharynx
- Metabolic: SIADH, hypothermia (1.7%)
- Anemia may be only manifestation; screen for hypothyroidism in pernicious anemia (Arch IM 1982;142:1465)

Cmplc: Myxedema coma (lethargy, confusion, psychosis, sometimes frontal/occipital headache) associated with severe infection, cold exposure, psychoactive meds (Geriatric Clin N Am 1993;222:279)

Lab:
- TSH > 10 mU/L; if TSH too costly, a T_4 > 8 pg/dL can rule it out; TSH may be increased by metoclopramide, dopamine blocker; there may be an acute elevation of TSH in nonthyroidal illness, recheck 4–6 wk after illness resolves; associated w elevated cholesterol
- R/o hypothalamic-pituitary axis damage: look for DI, acromegaly, hypogonadism, adrenal insufficiency
- If no sx, check antimicrosomal antibody; if increased, likely that subclinical hypothyroidism will convert within 5-yr period to clinical hypothyroidism

EKG: Sinus bradycardia, low-voltage, prolonged QT, AV block, intraventricular conduction delay

Xray: Pleural effusion

Rx:

Preventive: Screen women (U.S. Preventive Task Force, 1996) and men (= 2.5% subclinical; Arch IM 1990;150:785), low threshold for ordering in pts w nonspecific complaints (J Am Ger Soc 1996;44:50)

Therapeutic: L-thyroxine (Synthroid) 0.05 mg/d unless cardiac concerns; increase by 0.025 mg/d q 4–6 wk; in exceptional cases, eg, pts w heart disease may start as low as 0.0125 mg/d

Switching from desiccated thyroid preparation, which is variably bioavailable, to L-thyroxine may lead to iatrogenic hyperthyroidism

Hypothyroid pts with angina can undergo surgery without replacement; do not delay emergent CABG in hypothyroid patients with unstable angina; be careful of CNS-active meds that are cleared more slowly in hypothyroidism (Ann IM 1981;95:456; Am J Med 1984;77:261)

Thyroid replacement does not effect bone density

Myxedema coma: initial T_4 iv 100–1000 μgm; subsequent dose 100 μgm iv qd 1 through 10 d, then po

Pts w profound hypothyroidism requiring emergency general surgery should receive preoperative L-thyroxine 300–500 μgm slow iv infusion + hydrocortisone 300 mg iv; Swan-Ganz monitoring; watch for prolonged ileus and infection (altered febrile response)

Some argue if TSH mildly elevated and T_4 nl, treat to slow atherosclerosis and lower cholesterol (Solomen D, Intensive geriatric review course, UCLA, 1996)

HYPERTHYROIDISM

Clin Ger Med 1995;11:181; Jama 1995;273:808

Cause: Most common cause is toxic nodular goiter; Graves' or diffuse nodular goiter less common in late life; iatrogenic: takes T_4 5–6 half-lives to reach steady state in the elderly, or 6–7 wk in pts 80–90 yr old; therefore may induce hyperthyroidism if do not wait appropriate amount of time before increasing dose; T_4 may be suppressed in T_3 toxicosis (almost exclusively seen in the elderly); due to paucity of complaints, important to screen q 2 yr (w TSH) (J Am Ger Soc 1996;44:50)

Epidem: 15%–25% of cases occur in the elderly; 0.47% prevalence in community-based elderly

Pathophys: Apathetic thyrotoxicosis = diminished postreceptor responsiveness to thyroid hormone w age

Sx: Rarely report loose stools but may note a correction of constipation; reduction in appetite and consume less calories and weight loss; inability to rise from chair due to proximal muscle weakness; apathetic hyperthyroidism

Si: Tremor less common in elderly but when present is coarse, rather than fine as in younger patients; most frequent cardiac manifestation is sinus tachycardia

Cmplc: Accelerates bone turnover, leading to osteoporosis; causes insulin resistance (2%–3% of thyrotoxic pts develop clinically significant diabetes); CHF (60% of elderly persons w hyperthyroidism develop CHF); high-output failure leads to widened pulse pressure; 50% have Afib; 20% have angina (Nejm 1992;327:94); thyroid often largely substernal

Lab: TSH lowered by dopamine agonists and corticosteroids (Drinka P, Phoenix, AZ, 1997)

Xray: Diagnosis confirmed by increased uptake of radioactive iodine

Rx:

>   **Prevention:** If asx but TSH low w normal T_3, T_4, monitor more frequently for sx and increase in T_3, T_4 and if become present, treat
>
>   **Therapeutic:**
>   - ^{131}I for toxic multinodular goiter requires 2–3× the radioisotope dose for diffuse toxic goiter; for Graves': irradiation (Table 3-4), propylthiouracil (PTU) for 3 wk before radioactive iodine therapy to eliminate the possibility of radiation-induced thyroiditis;

Table 3-4. Radioisotope Use in Thyroid Disease

Iodine 131	Iodine 123	Technetium 99m
$t_{1/2}$ = 8d, 30% detection hyperactive thyroid, readily available, low cost, use to rx hyperthyroidism, thyroid cancer	$t_{1/2}$ = 13 h, 80% detection, not easily available, high cost	$t_{1/2}$ = 6 h, 90% detection, readily available, low cost, use to image thyroid when pt has had thyroid-blocking agents

Drugs that interfere w thyroid iodine absorption: adrenocorticosteroids, nitrates, PTU, ASA, sulfonamides, methimazole for 2 mo, myelogram contrast agent for 2 yr

major complication of radiation is hypothyoidism: 50% develop it within 20 yr

- Methimazole (Tapazole) when TSH low, T_3,T_4 normal but patient is sx (J Am Ger Soc 1996;44:573)
- Of Graves': β-blockers: for heat intolerance, anxiety, myopathy; adverse effects: cardiac, pulmonary, memory, mood, sleep disorders, fatigue

  PTU 100 mg or methimazole (Tapazole) 10 mg q 6–8 h blocks hormone synthesis; large goiters may require twice as much, rarely up to 1000 mg/d of PTU; euthyroid in 6 wk, then can begin maintenance 50–300/d × 1 yr; >one-third respond permanently; adverse effects include hypothyroidism, agranulocytosis (0.5%) (early in treatment, w large doses, reversible w withdrawal, baseline wbc and repeat w signs of infection—fever), skin rash, arthralgia, myalgia, neuritis, SLE, psychosis
- Of preop hyperthyroidism for emergency thyroid or nonthyroid surgery: iv loading dose of PTU 1000 mg or ipodate sodium 500 mg po × 5 d prior to surgery, or propranolol iv 1 mg/min during surgery

THYROID NODULES

Clin Ger Med 1995;11:291

Epidem: More frequent in elderly and more frequently malignant, and when malignant more aggressive than in younger patients; more common among women; differentiated tumors more aggressive at age >45 yr; anaplastic exclusively at age >65 yr

Sx: Dysphagia, pain suggest cancer

Si: Hard nodules, enlarged lymph nodes, rapid growth should raise suspicion of cancer

Crs: Variable and dependent on pathologic grade

Cmplc: Of multinodular goiter: thyrotoxicosis, subclinical thyrotoxicosis (Clin Endocrinol 1992;36:25), vocal cord paralysis, tracheal compression (Am J Med 1988;84:19)

r/o benign: colloid (60%), adenomas (30%); carcinoma (see Table 3-5), lymphoma frequently in persons w underlying Hashimoto's thyroiditis

Lab:

Pathologic: Fine-needle aspiration (FNA) bx—malignant reports in 5% of specimens, and an indication for surgery (except w lymphoma or anaplastic carcinoma); false-pos rate of 5%–7%; bx several areas of multinodular goiter (larger, harder ones, those that are cold on scan)

Xray: Both US and radionuclide scan more sens than palpation; nodules frequently cold and solid

Rx:

Therapeutic: Thyroid replacement: if TSH elevated, reassess nodule after 2 mo of thyroid replacement; multinodular goiters do not respond as well to suppressive therapy as Hashimoto's thyroiditis or simple diffuse goiters

Of hot nodules: older pts w hot nodules, nl T_4, but suppressed TSH (subclinical thyrotoxicosis) have increased risk for osteoporosis and possible underlying heart disease; should have lower threshold for radioactive rx

If benign FNA and nodule <2 cm, use suppression rx; if benign FNA and >2 cm, surgery indicated (larger nodules not as responsive)

Preoperative cardiac screening indicated for pts undergoing thyroid surgery w following risk factors: Q-wave MI on EKG, angina, DM, ventricular ectopy requiring rx, advanced age (Ann IM 1989;110:859)

THYROID CARCINOMA (Table 3-5)

Clin Ger Med 1995;11:271

Table 3-5. Thyroid Carcinoma

	Papillary	Follicular	Medullary	Anaplastic
Cause	Graves: LATS			
Epidem	75% of thyroid cancers	15%	5%	3%
Pathophys			Associated w MEN IIA, hyperparathyroidism, pheochromocytoma	
Sx	30% present as occult tumors; lymph node enlargement, hoarseness, dysphagia, neck pain	Slow-growing goiter; lymph node not as common as papillary; 50% metastatic at presentation; occasionally thyrotoxicosis		Sudden increase in size of goiter; difficulty breathing
Si	Bilateral		Mostly bilateral	Firm, tender w soft areas of hemorrhage, necrosis
Crs	Good prognosis if <1.5 cm despite lymph node involvement; 55% 10-yr survival; enters more malignant phase after 10 yr w. metastases to lung, bone (lytic), brain, and soft tissue	High mortality w vascular invasion	To lymph node liver, bone, adrenal	Mortality 6 mo to 1 yr
Lab	Psammoma bodies pathognomonic on histology		Calcitonin >250 pg/mL indicates cancer	
Rx	Surgery: total thyroidectomy w excision suspicious lymph nodes, ablate postoperatively w 131I; watch calcium levels postoperatively; f/u T4 q 6 mo, if elevated, check radioiodine scan and rx recurrent disease w 131I	Radioactive iocine; replace w T3 because shorter-acting and can discontinue for only 2 wk when checking radioactive thyroid scan yearly	Not responsive to radioiodine; rx w surgery	Radiation shrinks tumor (4–5000 rads); may cause tracheal obstruction; undifferentiated cancer fatal in 1 yr; rx doxorubicin (De Vita VT, Cancer principles and practice of oncology, 4th ed, Lippincott, 1993:1333)

LATS = long-acting thyroid stimulator; MEN = multiple endocrine neoplasia.
From Clin Ger Med 1995;11:271.

4. Neurology

STROKE

Cullison S, Seattle, Family practice review course, 3/95; Geriatrics 1992; 36:53; Am Fam Phys 1994;49:1777; Clin Ger Med 1993;9:705; Reuben DB, Ger Rev Syllabus Supplement 126S 1993; Am J Med 1996; 100:465; Circ 1996;94:1167; Arch Neurol 1995;52:347

Cause: Carotid or aortic arch (Nejm 1992;326:221), basilar system plaque and/or platelet emboli, cardiac emboli, vascular spasm, hypercoagulable states, and idiopathic

Risk Factors: HT, DM, CAD, MI, Afib (14% risk embolic stroke at onset and 5%/yr), peripheral vascular disease (PVD), smoking, lipids, homocysteinemia (Jama 1995;274:1526; Ann IM 1995;123:747; Nejm 1995;372:286,328; Jama 1997;227:1775)

Hemorrhagic Stroke: 50% are due to HT, 17% from amyloid angiopathy, 10% from anticoagulation rx, 5%–10% from brain tumors, 5% from smoking (Nejm 1992;326:1672; Curr Concepts Cerebro Dis 1990;25:31; 1991;26:1)

Epidem: 75% of pts w CVA are >75 yr; 2% incidence/yr for elderly; 35000 pts/yr in NH; 100 000/yr patients at home

Pathophys: Occasionally is vasospastic and can rx w calcium channel blocker (Nejm 1993;329:396) (Table 4-1)

Sx:

- TIA: most <24 h, 70% <1 h
- Infarct: h/o TIA (80%); nocturnal onset (60%)—early morning hours—awakens w stroke

  Anterior circulation sx: amaurosis fugax (Stroke 1990;21:201); weakness of arm > face > leg paresis (middle cerebral artery pattern); leg > arm > face paresis (anterior cerebral artery pattern); depression; abulia; delusions; aphasia if dominant hemisphere

Table 4-1. Stroke Types and Mortality

Cerebral Infarct (75%)	Intracerebral Hemorrhage (15%)	Subarachnoid Hemorrhage (10%)
40%	80%	50%

Posterior circulation sx: diplopia, numbness in face and mouth; slurred speech; loss of consciousness; crossed signs CN vs body; headache (HA); vomit; dizzy; ataxia

Lacunar: pure motor w internal capsule; pure sensory w thalamus; dysarthria and clumsy hand w pons, ataxia and hemiparesis w base pons; genu and internal capsule

- Embolism: 75% mid cerebral, 90% maximum loss at onset, loss of consciousness (LOC) common, seizure
- Hemorrhagic infarct: during physical activity, most commonly from berry aneurysm or microaneurysm from HT; decreased alertness, vomiting; hemiparesis w putamen or thalamus bleed; bilateral signs and coma w brainstem; HA, vertigo, ataxia, gaze, and facial palsy w cerebellar

Si:

- TIAs: in elderly, asx bruit present in 10% and does not correlate with CVA rate in or out of affected carotid distribution
- Infarct: specific occlusion patterns:
  Middle cerebral: face and arm motor; expressive aphasia (Broca's)
  Carotid watershed: parietal aphasias, weakness arm > face > leg
  Posterior cerebral: homonymous hemianopsia, hemisensory loss, memory loss (Curr Concepts Cerebro Dis 1986;21:25)
  Lateral medullary plate syndrome (posterior inferior cerebellar artery or PICA—Curr Concepts Cerebro Dis 1981;16:17): ipsilateral pain and temperature loss on face, contralateral for rest of body, hoarseness, swallowing dysfunction, Horner's, hiccoughs, ipsilateral cerebellar si's
  - Subarachnoid hemorrhage: HT, stiff neck
  - Cerebellar hemorrhage: awake, alert even with ophthalmoplegias; acute hypotonia; conjugate gaze paresis; skew deviation
  - Cerebral hemorrhage: seizure (13%) w onset or within 48 h
  - Brainstem hemorrhage: early loss of consciousness, brainstem si's, quadriplegia

NEUROLOGY

Crs:

- 20% of pts w TIAs will have CVA within 1 mo; 50% in 1 yr; 50% of pts w TIAs die of CAD while 36% die of CVA; association of TIA w MI as strong as MI and 3-vessel CAD (Am Fam Pract Series III Home study monograph 1995:195)
- Infarct: if there is even slightest voluntary twitch within 7 d of stroke onset, full upper extremity recovery may be expected; voluntary hip flexion pos predictor of ambulation, spasticity resolves, hyperreflexia persists
- Embolic stroke: 15% 30-d mortality; 12% of cardiac embolic stroke have 2nd embolus within 2 wk of first event
- Hemorrhagic stroke: over 1 mo one-third die, one-third are impaired, and one-third are OK (Nejm 1993;311:1547)

Cmplc:

- TIA: r/o migraine, subdural, hematoma, seizures, hypoglycemia, tumor, MS
- Stroke: r/o MI w EKG
- CVA: seizures, 33% of which occur within 2 wk after infarction; depression occurs in 40% of L-hemisphere infarctions; poststroke depression probably physiologic not psychological phenomenon (Stroke 1994;25:1099); periarthritis of shoulder after hemiplegia despite passive range of motion exercises; pulmonary emboli; pneumonias; UTIs

Lab:

Noninvasive: Carotid duplex US, carotid Doppler US, MRA all about 85% sens and 90% specif (Ann IM 1995;122:360; 1988; 109:805,835); CBC w platelets, PT/PTT; VDRL; EKG (r/o MI, arrhythmia), which often shows abnormal "anterior MI" patterns (Nejm 1974;291:1122; J Neur Surg 1969;30:521)

Hemorrhagic Stroke: LP preferably only after CT to r/o mass lesion; CSF: some intracerebral bleeds and all subarachnoid bleeds show grossly bloody tap w > 1000 rbc's/µL (100% sens, 80% specif), protein > 1 gm/dL; xanthochromia present in 90% (centrifuge immediately to avoid false-pos); rbc's decrease 10× from 1st to 3rd tube (80% sens, 60% specif) (Ann IM 1986; 104:880)

Xray: W/u TIA w US Doppler; CT best for acute bleed; MRI for lacunar—not good for acute bleed; old strokes not uncommonly found during acute episode by CT in elderly; MRI-A ? as good as angiography

Hemorrhagic Stroke: 25% of subarachnoid bleeds won't show blood on CT

Rx:

Preventive: Decrease systolic BP to 140 even in patients >80 yr; decreases long-term incidence of CVA by 30/1000 and MI by 55/1000; prefer thiazides and β-blockers, ACE inhibitors (for acute BP management, see treatment section)

Control blood sugar in diabetic patients

If smoke > 20 cigarettes/d, have 6× increased risk for CVA (Cullison S, Cerebral vascular disease, strokes and TIAs, at Family practice review course, Seattle, WA, 3/95); incidence falls significantly after 2 yr of not smoking and falls to risk of nonsmokers after 5 yr of not smoking

ASA after TIA reduces recurrence of nonfatal stroke, MI, and vascular death by 20%–25% (BMJ 1994;308:81,1540; Curr Opin Neurol 1994;7:48)

Warfarin for all Afib unless contraindications:

- Patients s/p MI w nonvalvular Afib (Nejm 1995;332:238)
- Patients w Afib and intrinsic heart disease, HT, LVH, previous TIA (Ann IM 1994;121:41,54); w recent cerebral ischemia: warfarin at INR = 2.0–3.0 (Nejm 1995;333:5; Jama 1995;274:1839)

Versus ASA for pts w nonvalvular Afib <60 yr, warfarin (Coumadin) for pts w nonvalvular Afib 65–75 yr, ASA for pts w nonvalvular Afib >75 yr (Lancet 1994;343:687)

Warfarin for patients w 60% carotid stenosis (Jama 1995;243:1421; Nejm 1995;332:238)

Therapeutic:

- TIA: endarterectomy if >70% stenosis (Nejm 325:445,1991; Jama 1995;273:1421); consider if combined cmplc rate of angiography and surgery at your hospital is <3%, since often morbidity is 14% in community hospitals, but only 1% in big centers; more risk of MI s/p endarterectomy in patients >70 yr old (Cardiovasc Surg 1993;1:30); ETT if any cardiac risk factors; warfarin × 3 mo course; if risk of bleeding, ASA 300 mg, if risk of bleeding ticlopidine (Ticlid) ? better (Med Let Drugs Ther 1992;34:65); adverse effects of ticlopidine: diarrhea, abdominal cramps, rarely neutropenia (monitor blood counts q 1 mo for 3–4 mo) (Ann IM 1994;121:45)

- Stroke in evolution: iv TPA within 3 h of onset of stroke results in 30% improvement in clinical outcome but increased incidence of intracranial hemorrhage within 36 h (6.45 vs 0.6%) (Nejm 1995;333:1581; Jama 1996;276:961), in patients up to 85 yr (Circ 1996;94:1826); alteplase (Activase) (Med Let Drugs Ther 1996;38:99)
- Nonhemorrhagic infarct: use anticoagulant only w CVA in evolution, TIA in pt on ASA or ticlopidine; otherwise risk of bleeding too great (American Heart Association, Stroke 1994;25:1901)

Acute Care (Curr Concepts Cerebro Dis 1989;24:1): Rx diastolic BP >140 or systolic >230 acutely with iv nitroprusside; if diastolic persists >105 or systolic >180 for 1–2 h, then rx with labetalol iv or po, mannitol 25–50 gm as 20% soln over 30 min q 3–12 h and/or furosemide iv, and/or nifedipine sl or po (sl nifedipine may lower BP too abruptly) (American Heart Association, Stroke 1994;25:1901); keep PCO_2 at 25–30 mmHg if on respirator; monitor; give 100–125 mL/h of Ringer's or D_5S

Supportive Care: Heparin sc to prevent DVT, which occurs in 70% (Ann IM 1992;117:353); poststroke depression: SSRIs (Stroke 1994;25:1099) or nortriptyline (Lancet 1984;1:297)

Follow-up Care:
- Embolic stroke: decreased by 86% if anticoagulate × 2 yr; annual bleeding rate 2.5% (Ann IM 1992;320:352,392), so maintain INR 2–3; warfarin if abnormal echocardiogram; anticoagulate >60% occluded asx carotid stenosis w intermittent or chronic Afib to decrease embolic stroke, NNT = 16 (Jama 1995; 273:1421); surgically fix >70% carotid stenosis (Nejm 1995; 332:238)
- Hemorrhagic infarct: prevent aspiration; hydration control; *don't lower BP;* supratentorial >5 cm size bad prognosis; pontine >3 cm bad prognosis

Rehab: Prognosis for patients w CVAs >65 yr: 10% no dysfunction, 40% moderate dysfunction, 40% severe dysfunction, 10% institutionalized; begin physical therapy right away after stroke w progression to full program as able; good prognostic signs: motivated to participate in rehab, follows one-step commands, memory to learn, bowel and bladder control, feeding and grooming skills, strong social support; successful rehab not associated w size of infarction or site of infarction (Arch Phys Med Rehab 1989;7:100) or age alone

6 mo to regain motor function w continuous gains for 2–3 yr, 2–3 yr to regain language function

Reimbursement from Medicare for rehab requires multidisciplinary approach, documentation of goals, documentation of improvement, goal cannot be maintenance

Criteria for admission to acute rehab facility: expected rapid rate of improvement, eg, 3–4 wk; tolerate 3 h/d of combined therapy 6–7 d/wk; minimal dementia; may want to use methylphenidate HCl (Ritalin) for severely depressed patients to ensure their candidacy for rehab but would try SSRIs first

To obtain rehab in the home, must need two therapies daily, as well as daily nursing and 24-h physician availability; location of rehab program may vary w managed-care programs

Team Management (poststroke rehab AHCPR Publc No. 95-0663, 1995)

Physical Therapy: Return of function 3 mo–1 yr: start brace when have "en masse" flexor or extensor synergism of all joints and 4/5 strength and can balance on good leg; then work on selective flexion and bed access; metal brace for spasticity

Shoulder pain common and has many possible causes: adhesive capsulitis; shoulder subluxation; rotator cuff injury; tenosynovitis; rarely reflex sympathetic dystrophy (cutaneous sensitivity and swelling of hand and arm); rx w range of motion exercises, hot and cold contrast baths; unresponsive, can try high-dose corticosteroids, stellate block; rx spasticity w baclofen, dantrolene, or tisanidine (D_2-adrenergic agonist not yet released on U.S. market), all of which cause sedation

Occupational Therapy: Diagnose and rx perceptual, cognitive losses, and ADL deficit, and help patient begin to engage in social activity again

Swallowing Evaluation (Table 4-2): 6 nerves and 25 facial and oral muscles involved; 40%–50% of stroke patients have some degree of dysphagia, which can carry up to a 40% risk of aspiration; transit time is measured by placement of examiner's index and third fingers at the top and bottom of the thyroid cartilage while patient swallows; delay >10 sec is associated w a significant risk of aspiration (Am Fam Phys 1994;49:1777); methylene blue dye test useful for patients w tracheostomy, dye in tracheal secretions after oral intake of dye in foods indicates aspiration (Am J Nurs 1995;95(8):34)

Table 4-2. Four Phases of Swallowing

Phase	Description	CN	Dysfunction	Assess
Oral preparatory	Lips closed, lubrication, chewing, tongue places bolus of food between tongue and palate	V, VII, XII, voluntary, cortical	Drooling, food pocketed on affected side, because no sensation	"Mi, mi, mi"
Oral	Food received into the pharynx beginning the reflex of swallowing	XII, voluntary, cortical	Coughing, choking	"La, la, la"
Pharyngeal	Tongue and pharynx walls push food into the esophagus, laryngeal elevation triggers closure of the epiglottis and vocal cords	IX, X, XI, involuntary, brainstem	Food stuck in throat, nasal regurgitation, coughing, choking, hoarseness	"Ga, ga, ga"
Esophageal	Upper esophageal sphincter closes, peristalsis moves food from esophagus to stomach	X, involuntary, brainstem		

From Am J Nurs 1995;95(8):34.

Feeding Recommendations:
1. 30-min rest before eating
2. Observation of eating essential until degree of risk established
3. Call button if eating without assistance
4. Allow 30–40 min for patient to eat meal
5. Juice better than water because taste helps locate food in mouth; the pulp in citrus juices may pose a problem
6. Avoid sticky, dry foods and mucus-producing foods such as milk products; just because patient has gag reflex does not mean will not aspirate; small amounts of food may not stimulate a gag reflex; may need to thicken fluids; chopped better than puree
7. Have pts clear their throat before swallowing, say "ah," and if sound is gurgly, may have aspirated; pt can perform finger sweep between swallows
8. Straws deposit food too far back in the throat; if patient has a weak swallow reflex, keep drinking glass three-fourths full so doesn't have to tilt head too far back
9. Keep patient upright 45–60 min after eating

PARKINSON'S DISEASE (Tables 4-3, 4-4)

Robbins L, UCLA, 1/96; Neurol 1994;44(suppl 10)

Cause: Environmental factors (African Americans have 5× risk of blacks in Nigeria); genetic cause chromosome 4 (Science 1996;274·1197); drug-induced Parkinson's in first 3 mo of therapy; drugs w antidopaminergic properties: haloperidol (Haldol), metoclopramide (Reglan), prochlorperazine (Compazine), amoxapine (Asendin), lithium, methyldopa (Aldomet)

Epidem: 50 000 new cases annually; 1/100 elderly vs 1/1000 general population; prevalence second only to Alzheimer's among degenerative neurologic diseases; cigarette smoking associated w decreased risk of Parkinson's (Neurology 1995;43:1041); NH patients w Parkinson's undertreated: lacking in physical therapy, rx of depression, adequate social interaction (J Am Ger Soc 1996;44:300; Nejm 1996;334:71)

Pathophys: Loss of pigmented neurons in substantia nigra and brain-

Table 4-3. Parkinson's Disease and Other Disorders

	Bradykinesia	Tremor	Automatic Dysfunction	Dementia	Depression	Vertical Gaze Paralysis/PDD	Other Neurologic Signs
Parkinson's 130/100 000	Facial Psychomotor slowing (cog wheeling) Slowed gait, decreased arm swing, forward flexion of neck and trunk Decrease turning (truncal rigidity) Decrease stride, step height (festonating gait) Drooling Hypophonic speech Micrographia	Alt. flexion ext fingers; resting, disappears with action; 4–8 c/sec; 70%	Hypotension Constipation (Shy-Drager) Increased salivation Increased sebum Dysphasia	40%; increased SE with meds	60%	Absent/absent	Absent
Supranuclear palsy	Axial rigidity Neck extension posture	Absent	Absent	Decreased cognition Decreased memory Decreased abstract thought	Present	Present/present	Absent

					Emotional lability		
Lacunar infarct:	Present	Absent	Present	—	Present	Absent/present	Present
Hypothyroid	Delayed response Slowed movement	Absent	Absent	Present	Present	Absent/absent	Present, cerebral dysfunction
Hypoparathyroid	Present	Absent	Absent	Absent	Absent	Absent/absent	Absent
Drugs	Present	May be present	Absent	Delirium	May be present	Absent/ absent	
Methyldopa							
Diazepam							
Lithium							
Reserpine							
Cholinergics							
Phenothiazines							
Excess vit B$_6$							
Other	Present	—	—	—	—	Absent/ absent	—
AIDS							
Neoplasia							
Trauma							
Jakob-Creutzfeldt							
Viral post-encephalitis							
Hydrocephalus							

Alt = alternating; ext = extension; SE = side effects; PPD = pseudobulbar dysarthria dysphagia.

Table 4-4. Clinical Classification of Tremors

Feature	Parkinsonian	Exaggerated Physiologic	Essential	Cerebellar
Frequency (Hz)	4–7	6–12	6–12	3–5
Amplitude	Coarse	Fine	Variable	Variable
Tremor at rest	++++	+	+	+
Tremor with action				
Postural	++	++++	+++	+++
Intention	++	++	++	++++
Distribution	Limbs, jaw, tongue	Limbs	Hands, head	Limbs, head

stem, Lewy bodies (concentric hyaline cytoplasmic inclusions); dopamine reduced in substantia nigra and corpus striatum; clinical symptoms when 80% depletion of striatal dopamine; neurotoxins: manganese toxicity, copper in Wilson's disease destroys dopaminergic neurons (Onion DK, The little black book of primary care, Blackwell Science, 1996)

Si (Table 4-5): Bradykinesia, rigidity (no loss of muscle strength), tremor (3–7 Hz), pill rolling tremor (?not as common in drug-induced Parkinson's or atherosclerotic Parkinson's) (Lancet 1984;2:1092; UCLA intensive review course, 1996), hypophonia, micrographia, depression 15%–40% (serotonin pathway may be affected too), drooling, constipation, seborrheic dermatitis

Crs: Average life expectancy = 12.3 yr, more rapid course in elderly, declining 5 yr after diagnosis; some live 20+ yr

Cmplc: Sleep disturbance common problem (J Am Ger Soc 1997;45: 194); drugs causing tremor: xanthines, β-agonists, valproate, heavy metals (Hg, Pb, As), thyroid, corticosteroids; multiple environmental toxins, methylphenyltetrahydropyridine (MPTP)

Table 4-5. Parkinson's Disease Age-related Characteristics

Older Pts (>65)	Younger Pts (<65)
Tremor (63%)	—
Bilateral (50%)	Unilateral (90%)
Difficulty walking (33%)	Stiff muscles (43%)

From Neurol 1988;38:1412.

R/o essential: is sporadic or hereditary w onset at early age; interferes w volitional movements, eg, writing, eating, highly skilled occupations; alcohol helps; β-blockers (propranolol 40–320 mg/d) significant improvement in one-half pts, primidone (Mysoline) (125–750 mg/d) also effective; clonazepam third choice

R/o: progressive supranuclear palsy (axial rigidity, vertical and later horizontal gaze paralysis, very little in the way of tremor)

Shy-Drager seen w bradykinesia, autonomic dysfunction, and cerebellar ataxia due to degeneration of sympathetic preganglionic nerves of thoracic and upper lumbar spinal cord, and not responsive to levodopa, hypotension resulting from rx of Parkinson's can be treated w high-salt diet or fludrocortisone

Lab: CBC, chem profile, albumin (nutritional assessment), thyroid profile, VDRL, Pb level

Xray: Chest xray—baseline for aspiration changes

Rx (Figure 4-1):

Therapeutic: Begin treatment when function is interfered with; Parkinson's disease fluctuates from hour to hour and day to day; therefore evaluate med adjustments over days to weeks, seek family, staff observations—entire 24-h periods

Selegiline (Deprenyl): MAO-B inhibitor may delay onset Parkinson's by 1–3 yr (Nejm 1989;321:1364); may not be so good for early Parkinson's (multicenter British study–BMJ 1995;311:1602); $1400–1500/yr; not active in gut so no tyramine effect; selegiline in doses of 2.5–10.0 mg/d blocks metabolism of CNS dopamine, thus enhancing levodopa; other newer agents may act in similar manner, eg, catechol O-methyltransferase (COMT) inhibitors; selegiline sometimes used in advanced disease for reducing wearing-off effect; adverse effects include insomnia, confusion, dyskinesias, gi distress, tricyclic antidepressants, selective serotonin reuptake inhibitors because of severe risk of hypertensive reaction, serious drug interactions w meperidine (Demerol), acts as MAO-A at >10 mg/d

Anticholinergics: generally toxic and minimally useful, benztropine 0.5 mg/d increasing slowly to 2 mg bid, trihexyphenidyl 2 mg/d increasing slowly to 5 mg tid; ethopropazine HCl (Parsidol) 50 mg/d gradually increasing to 600 mg/d for tremor

Amantadine: influences the release of dopamine; adverse effects: confusion, hallucinations, edema, livedo reticularis (purplish mottling of skin); modest short-lived efficacy; pts may respond again when reintroduced

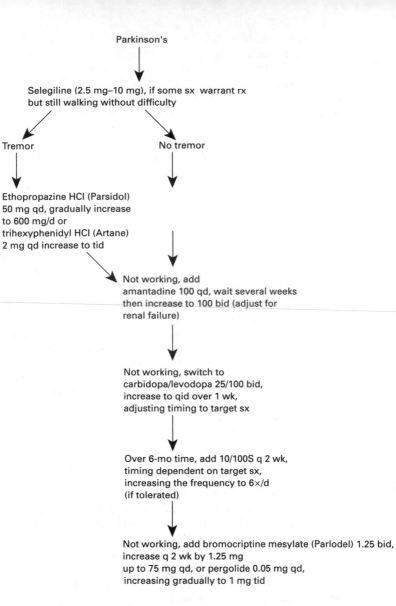

Parkinson's

↓

Selegiline (2.5 mg–10 mg), if some sx warrant rx
but still walking without difficulty

Tremor   No tremor

↓   ↓

Ethopropazine HCl (Parsidol)
50 mg qd, gradually increase
to 600 mg/d or
trihexyphenidyl HCl (Artane)
2 mg qd increase to tid

Not working, add
amantadine 100 qd, wait several weeks
then increase to 100 bid (adjust for
renal failure)

↓

Not working, switch to
carbidopa/levodopa 25/100 bid,
increase to qid over 1 wk,
adjusting timing to target sx

↓

Over 6-mo time, add 10/100S q 2 wk,
timing dependent on target sx,
increasing the frequency to 6×/d
(if tolerated)

↓

Not working, add bromocriptine mesylate (Parlodel) 1.25 bid,
increase q 2 wk by 1.25 mg
up to 75 mg qd, or pergolide 0.05 mg qd,
increasing gradually to 1 mg tid

Figure 4-1. Flow sheet for medications for Parkinson's disease.

Levodopa: effective, but because of adverse effects sometimes saved for more advanced disease, carbidopa/levodopa precipitates oxidation that further damages the substantia nigra and eventually spreads disease progression (J Am Ger Soc 1997;45:233), give w carbidopa (Sinemet) to limit breakdown (need at least 75–100 mg/d of carbidopa and do not exceed 200 mg/d); start with 25/100 one-half tab bid, increasing dose every week by one-half to 1 tab daily (2–8 tabs/d = $51–$205/mo); levodopa requirement for most pts is 500–1000 mg; therefore may need to add 10/100 mg tabs ($60/tab/mo) to increase levodopa but keep down carbidopa; painful dystonia upon awakening is a good indication that levodopa should be increased; give 2nd dose in afternoon to avoid insomnia; major side effects: hallucinations, psychosis; dyskinesias usually mean there is too much dopamine; take controlled release (CR) with food, and increase total dose of levodopa by 30% because not as bioavailable as short-acting (Nejm 1993;329:1021), CR 50/200 mg tid or qid; combine CR night with multiple small doses during day, 25/100 mg CR (2–8 tabs/d = $41–$163/mo); use 50/100 mg CR for motor fluctuations (2–6 tabs/d = $85–$254/mo) (Am Fam Phys 1996;53:1281); consider cisapride to help w absorption if levodopa ineffective; Diphenide for nausea (doesn't block dopamine receptors as other antinausea medications do) (chlorperazine, metaclopramide); avoid supplements that contain high doses of B-6 (50–100 mg B-6) because reduces activity of carbidopa; transdermal levodopa under investigation (Nejm 1993;329:1021)

Dopamine agonists: may want to start rx w dopamine agonist to delay or minimize use of carbidopa/levodopa, and also to avoid anticholinergic drugs; don't need to avoid protein in diet because doesn't affect absorption of dopamine

Bromocriptine (Parlodel) at 20–30 mg moderate effects on bradykinesia, can be added to levodopa to reduce the dose needed of levodopa, start at 1.25 and increase over several days to weeks (every week by 1.25–2.50-mg/d increments); side effects: nausea, vomiting, dry mouth, orthostasis, confusion hallucinations; ropinirole and pranipexole not expected to have side effects of bromocriptine, alter overall symptomatic course of PD

Antioxidants (vit E), selegiline might help

Pergolide (Permax) when bromocriptine not effective, both expensive

NEUROLOGY

(Mayo Clin Proc 1988;63:969); pergolide better (Neurol 1995;45: 522)

High drug costs and variable drug effectiveness over time mandate regular reviews, including trials off drugs, with careful, comprehensive, detailed observations to ascertain drug effectiveness or ineffectiveness

Muscle relaxants for pain and cramping

Clozapine (Clozaril) for hallucinations so can keep on using levodopa and selegiline

Stereotactic pallidotomy: long-term risks/benefits not established, complications include visual field deficits, contralateral paralysis, and speech problems (Med Let Drugs Ther 1996;38:107)

Fetal cell transplantation: postop sleep disturbance and mental status change more common and profound in older pts (Ann Neurol 1988;24;150)

PO tremor may be coexistent with familial tremor—propranolol-responsive (20–320 mg) (Arch Neurol 1986;43:42); high dosing may worsen depression and sleep disturbance

Depression responsive to nortriptyline—mild anticholinergic effects, also helps movement disorder, sialorrhea, tremor; serotonin reuptake inhibitors helpful as well, but have also been known to cause akathisia (β-blockers rx of choice for this side effect); both tricyclics and serotonin reuptake inhibitors can cause myoclonus, which can be controlled w clonazepam; identify and monitor specific "target" depression sx; may not require "chronic" antidepressants—review useful

Seborrheic dermatitis may be relieved by levodopa, ketoconazole (Nizoral) plus careful attention to hygiene

Team Management: Restricted protein diet—limit to protein meal at dinner time; investment in long-term work w family and staff education vital to quality management

SEIZURES

Nurs Home Med 1995;3:4b; Nejm 1990;323:1468

Cause: In 85%–90% of new-onset seizures, there is identifiable brain lesion; vascular disease 50% of time (one-third occur w onset embolic event, one-third occur during rehab phase, one-third are recurrent); focal seizure usually caused by brain tumor (cause of seizures in 12% of elderly population), brain abscess, previous head trauma; generalized seizure associated w h/o meningitis, encephalitis; 25% of pts w late-stage Alzheimer's have generalized seizures; metabolic; hypoxia

Epidem: Occur 2–3× more frequently than in younger pts; complex partial seizures common; fewer than 20% of *NH* pts on anticonvulsants actually have a seizure diagnosis (Nurs Home Med 1995;3:4b)

Sx: "Don't feel myself, something's happening"

Si:

- Generalized tonic-clonic motor (grand mal) most common type of seizure in elderly
- Complex partial sz: "tune out": intermittent confusion, disorientation, staring; repetitive motor acts: patting, rubbing, smacking lips, rarely wandering, or disrobing

Cmplc: Fractures, states of confusion, aspiration pneumonia

R/o early dementia or late dementia behaviors can be confused w partial complex seizures; focal seizures can be confused w TIAs

Lab: No LP unless suspect meningitis

Noninvasive: EEG if confusing differential

Xray: MRI best for small structural lesions

Rx:

Therapeutic (Table 4-6): Because of high rate of recurrence of seizure in old people, should start antiepileptic drug after first seizure unless obvious metabolic cause (Lancet 1988;1:721); adverse effects of neuroleptics: gait disturbance, sedation, tremor; folate deficiency predisposes pts to neurotoxicity

Carbamazepine (Tegretol): for focal seizures, 100 mg bid–tid; anticholinergic sides effect; pts with heart block can have conduction abnormalities; induces cytochrome P-450 system, so interacts with drugs metabolized with this system, eg, antidepressants, can cause hyponatremia, neutropenia

NEUROLOGY

Table 4-6. Anti-Convulsant Drugs					
	Carbamazepine	Phenytoin	Valproate	Gabapentin	Lamotrigine
Protein-bound (%)	75	90	95	0	55
Half-life (h)	12	24	12	5–8	30
Level (ng/mL)	6–12	10–25	50–150	>5	>2

Valporate: for generalized seizures, 250 mg bid–3 gm/d, inhibits hepatic drug-metabolizing enzymes so raises levels of benzodiazepines; pts may develop increased bleeding time; gi side effects

In pts w long-standing epilepsy on phenobarbital (>60 mg not usually tolerated, resulting in severe mental, behavioral effects, may also get osteopenia secondary to altered vit D metabolism) or phenytoin (Dilantin, 200–400 mg usual dose), drug need not be changed unless experiencing side effects (hirsutism, gum hyperplasia, folate deficiency, osteopenia secondary to impaired calcium absorption)

(Phenytoin level × 4.4)/pt's serum albumin
= effective phenytoin level

The lower the albumin, the more free drug fraction, the higher the effective level of phenytoin; therefore NH pts usually have a 25%–50% higher "effective" phenytoin level than reported

Neuroleptics, especially phenothiazines/antidepressants, lower seizure threshold, especially w h/o alcoholism

CNS stimulants such as methylphenidate (Ritalin), pemoline (Cylert), oral decongestants, pentoxifylline (Trental), theophylline can provoke seizures (Nurs Home Med 1995;3:4b)

Enteral feedings, milk, supplements, and antacids reduce absorption of phenytoin and should be spaced several hours apart

Diarrhea can reduce the amount of anticonvulsant or any drug absorbed via the oral route

Consider discontinuation of seizure med if long seizure-free period and normal EEG (Ger Rev Syllabus Suppl 1994;1:127S)

Gabapentin (Nejm 1996;334:1583; Neurol 1994;44:787) (GABA agonist) for partial seizures, lipid-soluble; doesn't affect concentrations of other seizure meds

Lamotrigine (Lamictal, a phenyltriazine derivative)—decrease the dose if given w other seizure meds (Nurs Home Med 1996;4:6b)

Some advantages to newer drugs: less drug interaction; lamotrigine single daily dose, less ataxia, and cognitive impairment

Team Management: Educate family and staff on recognition and responses

SLEEP PROBLEMS

Am Fam Phys 1994;51:191; Alessi C, Geriatric Intensive Review Course UCLA 1/96

Cause: Transient: stress, new bed, change time zone; chronic: depression, anxiety, substance abuse, pain, paresthesia, dyspnea, GE reflux, fear of death, delirium, myoclonus, sleep apnea; drugs: alcohol, antihypertensives, antineoplastics, β-blockers, caffeine, diuretics, levodopa, nicotine, oral contraceptives, phenytoin (Dilantin), serotonin reuptake inhibitors, protriptyline (Vivactil), corticosteroids, stimulants, theophylline, thyroid hormone

Types:

1. Difficulty initiating or maintaining sleep (insomnia or dyssomnias)
2. Excessive sleep
3. Sleep-wake cycle problems
4. Parasomnias occurring during sleep-wake transitions; characterized as behaviors that intrude into sleep but do not change sleep architecture, eg, nocturnal leg cramps

- Sleep disorders associated w Alzheimer's: increased duration, increased frequency of awakenings; decreased REM, stages 3 and 4 sleep; daytime napping; sleep apnea in later stages
- Sleep disorders associated w depression: more nighttime wakefulness and decreased slow-wave sleep; early morning awakening; more REM sleep earlier in night; ?community-dwelling elderly have decreased latency (number of minutes to fall asleep)
- Sleep apnea: repeated cessations for ≥ 10 sec w oxygen saturation ≤ 80%

Central: simultaneous cessation of breathing effort and nasal and oral airflow, as well as cessation of effort by diaphragm muscles

Obstructive: airflow stops while thoracic respirations persist (Sci Am 1996;11(13))

Mixed: (features of both) most common

- Periodic leg movements: characterized by debilitating, repetitive, stereotypic leg movements occurring in non-REM sleep
- Restless leg syndrome: uncontrollable urge to move one's legs at night, "creepy-crawling" sensation

Epidem: 50% of community have sleep problems; 90% of *NH pts;* 70%

of caregivers cited sleep problems as reason for admitting relatives to NH; NH residents awake on average q 20–25 min during the night; psychoactive meds dampen normal diurnal variation in sleep, eg, sleep during day, not at night

Increased mortality when oxygen saturation <85% and >20 episodes apnea/night

Pathophys: Normal changes in sleep pattern with age: sleep latency increased; sleep efficiency decreased (ratio of time asleep to time in bed); earlier bedtime; earlier morning awakening; more arousals during night; more daytime napping

Changes in sleep structure w age:
- Total REM sleep decreases
- Earlier-onset REM, and it does not increase in duration throughout the night as in young people
- Stages 1 and 2 (light sleep) remain the same
- Stages 3 and 4 (deep sleep, slow high-amplitude delta-wave sleep) decreased

Sx: Loss of concentration and memory, dysphoria, malaise, irritability, daytime napping, fatigue, interference w ADLs, headaches on awakening

Si: Sleep apnea: consider if pt has unexplained right-sided heart failure, decreased cognitive function; most severe episodes occur in REM sleep

Compl: Pulmonary HT, RV failure

Lab:

    Noninvasive: Indications for polysomnography in a sleep laboratory: sleep apnea, narcolepsy, periodic leg movements

Rx:

    Preventive:
- Screening questions: Is pt satisfied w his/her sleep? Does sleep or fatigue intrude w daytime activities? Does bed partner notice snoring, interrupted breathing, leg movements?
- Sleep hygiene: bed at same time each night; bedroom environment conducive; avoid excessive napping or before bedtime exercise; exercise helps (Jama 1997;277:32), exercise no help w sleep in NH setting (J Am Ger Soc 1995;43:1098); comfortable levels—temperature, light, noise; if can't get to sleep in one-half hour, get out of bed and participate in nonstimulating activity and return to bed when sleepy; light snack; relaxation techniques

Table 4-7. Benzodiazepines—Onset and Elimination Characteristics

Elimination	Fast Onset	Intermediate Onset	Slow Onset
Fast (6 h)	Zolidem (Ambien) Zolpidem	Triazolam (Halcion), oxazepam (Serax)	—
Intermediate (15 h)		Lorazepam (ativan), alprazelam (Xanax)	Temazepam (Restoril)
Slow (30–72 h)	Diazepam (Valium), clorazepate (Tranxene)	Chlordiazepoxide (Librium), flurazepam (Dalmane), clonazepam (Klonopin)	Prazepam (Centrax)

From Med Let 1996;38:60.

for those who ruminate; light therapy if a symptom of seasonal affective disorder (Jama 1997;277:990)

Therapeutic (Table 4-7):

- Chronic insomnia: intermittent dosing (2–4× weekly) (Nejm 1997;336:341)
- Most OTC hypnotics are antihistamines w sedating properties; they also have anticholinergic properties and should be discouraged in the elderly
- If elderly pt on low-dose barbituates, glutethimide, or chloral hydrate for years, may be reasonable to continue if pt very resistant to stopping it or may need to consult w psychiatrist (Ger Rev Syllabus 1996;175)
- Sedating antidepressants such as doxepin, amitriptyline (Elavil), and trazodone may help w sleep, especially w underlying depression, bruxism, and fibromyalgia
- Choral hydrate/hypnotics for 2–4 wk, become tolerant, consider every 3 nights to avoid tolerance; gradual tapering rather than abrupt discontinuation following prolonged use of agent (Drugs 1993;45:44)
- Benzodiazepines: work on GABA pathway, highly protein-bound; highly lipid-soluble; active metabolites prolonged in obese pts, except oxazepam (Serax) and lorazepam (Ativan) which are altered to inactive metabolites; many undergo oxidative hepatic metabolism: alprazelam (Xanax), chlordiazepoxide

(Librium), clorazepate (Tranxene), diazepam (Valium), prazepam (Centrax); levels are increased by meds that inhibit liver metabolism: cimetidine, contraceptives, disulfiram, fluoxetine (Prozac), INH, valproic acid

- Clonazepam (Klonopin) for nocturnal myoclonus
- No flurazepam (Dalmane); has long half-life (85 h); accumulates; don't use in elderly
- Temazepam (Restoril), effective for 6–8 h but has 2–3-h onset
- Triazolam (Halcion) psychosis and violent behavior in doses over 1 mg (maximum dose prescribed = 0.5)
- Quazepam (Doral) has a metabolite w a long half-life (72 h)
- Zolpidem (Ambien) not a benzodiazepine, no anticonvulsant or myorelaxant properties; as yet very little in the way of side effects reported: no withdrawal effects, no rebound insomnia, no tolerance; effects last a year; rapid onset; lasts 2–4 h; can use w warfarin; start at 5-mg dose (cognitive impairment at higher doses); fewer falls; twice as expensive as triazolam (Halcion); side effects: nightmares, agitation, headache, dizziness, daytime drowsiness, impaired memory and unsteady gait in the middle of the night (J Clin Psychopharmacol 1993;13.100)
- When withdrawing from short-acting benzodiazepines, decrease drug by 50% first week, and then by one-eighth for each of the next 4–8 wk
- Alleviation of insomnia w timed exposure to bright light (J Am Ger Soc 1993;41:829)
- Melatonin po 2 mg improves sleep efficiency 75%–85% (Lancet 1995;346:541)
- Chloral hydrate 500 mg, tolerance, increases warfarin metabolism

Of obstructive sleep apnea: tricyclic antidepressants reduce REM sleep and therefore ameliorate apnea; progesterone helps by increasing respiratory drive (Nejm 1990;323:520); dental prostheses; tracheotomy

CPAP (5–20 cm H_2O 50%–70% successful) for central and mixed sleep apnea

Of nocturnal myoclonus: avoid caffeine, tricyclics; clonazepam 0.25 mg hs increasing by 0.25 mg q 2 wk to maximum of 2 mg, trazodone 50–150 mg hs, levodopa 100–200 mg, carbamazepine

Of restless leg syndrome: avoid caffeine, tricyclics, antipsychotics, antihistamines; vit E 800–1200 IU/d, quinine, levodopa, or dopamine agonist antiparkinsonian drug, cautious use of narcotic analgesics

---

NEUROLEPTIC MALIGNANT SYNDROME (NMS)

Med Clin N Am 1993;77:185

Cause: Idiosyncratic reaction involving dopamine blockade, neuroleptic-induced hyperthermia via dysregulation of hypothalamus and basal ganglia; and muscle rigidity related to myonecrosis (Med Clin N Am 1993;77:185)

Epidem: Rare with incidence 0.02%–3.23%; risk factors: increased age, high-dose–high-potency neuroleptics such as haloperidol, thiothixene, fluphenazine, and trifluoperazine; may also see increased incidence with depot meds, lithium, antidepressants or multiple neuroleptics (low dose, low potency), carbidopa/levodopa, and withdrawal of amantadine; increased incidence in pts with h/o NMS, dehydration, lyte imbalance, thyrotoxicosis, and elevated ambient temperature (Med Clin N Am 1993;77:185); elderly particularly at risk because of underlying CNS impairment which can predispose them to NMS (J Am Ger Soc 1996;44:474)

Pathphys: Precipitated by any med that acts as D_2 dopamine receptor antagonist; severe dopamine blockade–induced parkinsonism with resulting muscle rigidity, then myonecrosis; autonomic thermogenic dysregulation via dopaminergic imput also postulated (Dis Nerv Syst Clin Neurobiol 1992;62:831)

Si: Hyperthermia w diaphoresis occurs in 98% of pts, but can be lacking in elderly; rigidity 97%; other movement disorder changes less often; mental status changes vary from clouded consciousness to coma; 97% pts autonomic instability, tachycardia, hypotension; tachypnea occurs secondary to metabolic acidosis, pneumonia, or pulmonary embolism (Med Clin N Am 1993;77:185; Clin Pharmacol Ther 1991;50:580)

Crs: High mortality if untreated; 10%–20% mortality with treatment; usually occurs soon after initiating neuroleptic treatment or with dose increases; recovery usual within 10 d, 97% by 30 d (Med Clin N Am 1993;77:185)

Cmplc: Cerebellar or other brain damage secondary to hypothermia;

fatal arrhythmias, metabolic acidosis, pulmonary emboli, pneumonia, and respiratory arrest

R/o encephalopathies, tumors, CVA, seizures, infections, endocrinopathies (thyrotoxicosis, pheochromocytoma), SLE, heat injury, toxins, drugs (Med Clin N Am 1993;77:185; Psych Ann 1991;21: 130)

Lab: EKG, CBC (leukocytosis common), CPK elevations at times extremely high; r/o hypothyroid, polymyositis, mesenteric vascular occlusion, rheumatoid arthritis, cancer of prostate, colon, lung (small cell), chronic renal disease; myoglobinuria (67%); LDH, transaminases, and aldolase may also be elevated from myonecrosis; metabolic acidosis and hypoxia may be present

Rx: Discontinue all neuroleptics and other centrally acting antidopaminergics, cardiac monitoring; bromocriptine 7.5–60.0 mg daily po or via NG tube; dantrolene, initially 1–2 mg/kg iv, then 10 mg/kg daily, may have synergistic effect; other useful meds: amantadine, benzodiazepines to lessen agitation; electroconvulsive therapy for refractory cases, but can also lead to NMS when given to pts exhibiting extrapyramidal adverse effects

Team Management: Alert to observe carefully for early signs in elderly when using highest-risk drugs (neuroleptics)

5. Psychiatry

DEPRESSION

Nejm 1989;320:164; Am J Ger Psychiatry 1993;1:421; 1994;2:193

Cause: Often situational (losses, illness, family stress, caregiver stress); hypothalamic-pituitary-adrenal axis and circadian rhythm disruption; hypokalemia, hyponatremia, MI, COPD, pernicious anemia, cancer, stroke involving left or right hemisphere, especially those close to the frontal pole (Aging 1994;6:49); drugs including alcohol, amantadine, antipsychotics, cimetidine (within several weeks of beginning therapy), clonidine, cytotoxic agents, digoxin, α-methyldopa (occurs w higher doses, mild, occurring within weeks of initiation of drug and lasts several weeks after cessation of drug), propranolol, sedatives, steroids, reserpine (may be severe w suicidal behavior and sometimes does not clear w cessation of reserpine, necessitating antidepressant therapy or ECT) (Jenike MA, Geriatric psychiatry and psychopharmacology, Mosby–Year Book, 1989)

Epidem: Prevalence is 10%–15% in the geriatric population, 8%–10% in nonagenarians (Br J Psychiatry 1995;167:61); 3rd leading cause of injury-related death in the elderly (Mmwr 1996;45:3); major depression increases risk for MI (Circ 1996;943:3123); major depression 1%–2% of elderly patients, minor depressions still cause substantial morbidity

Pathophys: MAO activity is increased in brains of elderly (Am J Psychiatry 1984;141:1276)

Sx: Careful hx is key to dx; 2 wk of depressed mode and 4/8 of following for major depression: impaired sleep often w early morning awakening (depressed pts have more rapid onset of REM sleep than normal elderly pts), decreased interest in usual sources of pleasure (anhedonia), feelings of guilt, decreased energy, altered concentration, and/or decreased appetite, psychomotor retardation or agitation, suicidal ideation; late-life depression is more associated with medical, neurologic illness, and dementia (DSM IV); less guilt, more somatic complaints (Small GW, Intensive Geriatric Review Course, UCLA, 1996); always ask directly about depressed mood; present elderly cohorts may resist dx because of sense of shame or self-blaming

Masked depression may present as somatization syndrome and pts may deny depression when asked (J Am Ger Soc 1995;43:216); atypical presentations: hypochondriasis, pain syndromes, delusions, shoplifting, alcoholism, depressive dementia, malnutrition, passive suicide, anxiety/agitation (J Am Ger Soc 1989;37:458); watch especially for depression as earliest presentation of mild cognitive losses of Alzheimer's

Psychotic depression: delusions more common than hallucinations, themes of guilt, hypochondriasis, nihilism, persecution and jealousy, different from delusions of dementia where pts not sad, usually think people are stealing things

Bipolar illness in the elderly: paranoid delusions, circumferential speech; may be as many as 10 yr between first depressive and manic episode; predominance of depressive symptoms; irritability and anger more common; greater duration of episodes, mortality rate higher for bipolar than unipolar

Rapid cycling more common in elderly women on antidepressants or with thyroid disease: 4 or more distinct episodes of mania, hypomania, or depression within a 12-mo period (Calabreese JR, Diagnosis of bipolar disorder and its subtypes, in Bipolar disorder, Keystone, CO, 1993:12)

Si: Depression scales (J Psych 1983;17:37); weight loss; association of low diastolic BP and depressive symptoms in community-dwelling elderly men (BMJ 1994;308:446)

Crs: Relapse rate is increased (19%) compared to younger (J Am Ger Soc 1987;35:516; Convuls Ther 1989;5:75); poorest prognosis: recent bereavement, delusions (as commonly as 50% of the time in the elderly), panic disorders; decreased heart rate variability increases risk for cardiac mortality and morbidity in depressed CAD pts (Am J Cardiol 1995;76:562)

Cmplc: Suicide—20% fatal

R/o grief reaction (beginning within 3 mo of loss and lasting a year), dysthymia (not free of depression for >2 mo over a 2-yr period, secondary dysthymia in the elderly results from chemical depen-

Table 5-1. Tricyclic Levels

Levels Increased by	Levels Decreased by
Aging	Smoking
Weight loss	Hyperlipidemia
Inflammatory disease	Barbiturates
Antipsychotics	Anticholinergics
Increased urine pH	Decreased urine pH
Morphine sulfate	
Cimetadine	
Steroids	

dency, anxiety, stress, and physical illness), schizophrenia (bizarre delusions and hallucinations), drug reactions

Lab:

Chemistry: TSH, B_{12} level, lytes, CBC; most reliable drug levels obtained 12 h after last dose w the following meds: imipramine (therapeutic level = 125 ng/mL), desipramine (therapeutic level = 225 ng/mL), nortriptyline (therapeutic level = 150 ng/mL) (Am J Psychiatry 1985;142:155) (Table 5-1)

Rx:

Medications:

General Considerations: Agitated depression responds less well than melancholic (vegetative) depression

Use one-third usual adult doses (demethylation is decreased in the elderly), increase monthly, and use smallest effective dose for maintenance therapy

Biologic symptoms improve before mood (insomnia in first few days)

Familial response good predictor of individual success w an antidepressant

Administer 3–4 h before bedtime except w trazodone (Desyrel absorbed rapidly)

Only prescribe 1 gm of tricyclic antidepressants (TCAs) at a time to avoid overdose (2 gm w trazodone)

May discontinue antidepressant after 6 mo if no previous episode of depression in 2½ yr, reduce the dose by one-half, then taper by 25 mg/wk to avoid cholinergic hyperactivity w abrupt withdrawal (malaise, chills, muscle aches, coryza); maintenance doses of antidepressants should be as high as doses for acute treatment; if seasonal affective disorder (SAD) pattern, take into consideration when planning discontinuation

Avoid tertiary amine tricyclics because of increased anticholinergic side effect (Mayo Clin Proc 1995;70:999), and potent α-blocker activity producing postural hypotension (may not improve w dose reduction); except in the following situations:

Imipramine (Tofranil) up to 150 mg po qd in pts w depression and urge incontinence

Amitriptyline (Elavil) up to 75 mg po qd in poststroke depression and pseudobulbar crying

Doxepin (Sinequan) in pts w PUD (doxepin is somewhat less sedating than the other tertiary amines and is a potent histamine antagonist)

Chlomipramine (Anafranil) up to 75 mg po qd for obsessive-compulsive disorder

Secondary Amine Tricyclics: Have less anticholinergic side effect but beware of additive effects w other anticholinergic meds (even at therapeutic doses) producing anticholinergic syndrome (anxiety, confusion, assaultive behavior), paranoia, hallucinations, which can lead to coma and death; drugs w anticholinergic side effect include antispasmodics, antidiarrheal agents, low-potency antipsychotics, antiparkinsonian meds, antihistamines, drugs for vertigo, and OTC sleep meds; tricyclics block effects of clonidine (Catapres) (American College of Psychiatrists, Update Psychotr Drug Interact 1993;13:1); quinidine and carbamazepine (Tegretol) increase tricyclic levels; tricyclics cause more impotence while SSRIs cause more anorgasmia; tricyclics can cause mania (Am J Psychiatry 1995;152:1130)

Nortriptyline (Pamelor, Avantyl) 10–35 mg po qd, higher plasma concentrations correlate w greater cognitive impairment (Drugs Aging 1994;5:192); least hypotensive effects

Desipramine (Norpramin) 25–150 mg po qd; useful if sleeping too much (less sedating than "snortriptyline"), not as effective in the elderly (J Clin Psychopharmacol 1995;15:99)

Treatment of TCA overdose: recognize anticholinergic side effects of excitation/restlessness w paradoxical progressive sedation, tonic-clonic seizure, flushed-dry skin, pupils dilated, bowel sounds decreased, urinary retention, tachyarrhythmias, hypotension

QRS > 0.10 sec predictive of life-threatening ventricular arrhythmia

and seizure (Nejm 1985;313:474); R wave on aVR >3 mm best
predictive value for seizure or ventricular arrhythmia (Ann EM
1995;26:196)

Treat cardiac arrhythmias w propranolol; avoid digoxin, procaine,
physostigmine; monitor for several days

Initial therapy: can't remove w hemodialysis because protein-bound;
pills radiopaque; lavage w charcoal (effective for a prolonged time
after overdose because of paralytic ileus due to overdose), alkalin-
ize urine w sodium bicarbonate

SSRIs: Increasingly replacing tricyclics because of low side effect
profiles in the elderly (AJGP 1996;4:S51), but are not as effective
as tricyclics in melancholic elderly hospitalized pts (Am J Psychiatry 1994;151:1735); not sedating, don't produce anticholinergic
side effects, are not cardiotoxic and do not produce hypotension;
useful in obsessive-compulsive disorder, panic attacks as well;
may cause overstimulation and worsen anxiety sx, but are being
used in low doses for anxiety; not effective in neuropathic pain
(Nejm 1992;326:1250); $60/mo; more sexual dysfunction than
other antidepressants (Geratrics 1995;50:S-41), pseudoparkinson-
ism and inappropriate secretion ADH are also frequent side
effects

Fluoxetine (Prozac): half-life = 3 d, 10 mg po qod–20 mg po qd,
increase q 2–4 wk; takes 5 wk to washout before adding MAO
inhibitor; potent inhibitor of cytochrome P-450, thereby increasing
concentrations of cyclic antidepressants, class Ic antiarrhythmics,
β-blockers, calcium channel blockers, chlorpromazine (Thorazine),
risperidone (Risperdal), carbamazepine (Tegretol), phenytoin
(Dilantin), astemizole (Hismanal), terfenadine (Seldane) (Psychiatry
Drug Alerts 1996;10(9):65); can give trazodone (Desyrel) 25 mg
or clonazepam (Klonopin) 0.5 mg hs for insomnia (Am J Psychiatry 1994;151:1069); serotonin syndrome from combination of fluoxetine and trazodone (Psychosom 1995;36:159); 5% gi side
effect or headache; more anxiety, nervousness, anorexia than other
SSRIs (J Clin Psychiatry 1994;55:S10); mania in 1% general population on SSRIs, and more common in bipolars; paranoia, psychosis; extrapyramidal occasionally (Nejm 1994;371:1354); skin rash

Sertraline (Zoloft): half-life = 25 h, 25 mg po qod and up to 125 mg
qd in 1–2 wk, 14-d washout before giving MAO inhibitor;
increases warfarin, diazepam, tolbutamide, tegretol; not sedating;
can produce nausea and diarrhea

Paroxetine (Paxil): half-life = 24 h, 10 mg po qd; increases digoxin, tricyclics; the most sedating of the SSRIs; produces constipation, headache, and sexual dysfunction equally as much as other SSRIs

Fluvoxamine (Luvox): half-life = 15 h, most rapid onset of the SSRIs, 50 mg po qd; least effect on cytochrome P-450 D6 but more on P-450 3A4; increases propranolol, warfarin, theophylline (P-450 1A2), carbamazepine, tricyclics, haloperidol (Haldol), phenytoin, caffeine, alprazolam, triazolam, nonsedating antihistamines, eg, terfenadine, astemizole; gi side effects more pronounced than sexual dysfunction or headache

Serotonin Agonists: Much more sedating than SSRIs and therefore are used in settings where sedation is required as in agitated depression; cytochrome Pu isoenzyme inhibition and drug interaction (AFP 1997;55:1692)

Trazodone (Desyrel): not as effective as other antidepressants; dose 50 mg up to 150 mg po qd; no interactions w MAO inhibitors; increases digoxin levels; significant hypotension, as well as nausea and vomiting

Nefazadone (Serzone): up to 50 mg po bid, increase q 1–2 wk; up to 300 mg bid, inhibits cytochrome P-450 3A4 and decreases clearance of triazolam, alprazolam, antihistamines; not interactive w MAO inhibitors; less sedating than trazodone; some anorgasmia

Mirtazopine (Raveron) 15 mg q Hs—not interact w other medications

Bupropion (Dopaminergic): 50 mg tid up to 100 tid, divided doses obviate seizures; not sedating; may use trazodone, clonazepam for insomnia as w fluoxetine; no MAO inhibitor interactions; no cardiotoxicity; may exacerbate preexisting HT, no sexual dysfunction or headache; extrapyramidal side effects uncommon

Amoxapine (Asendin): Metabolite of loxapine, which is an antipsychotic; 25 mg po hs; has a methylphenidate-like effect on appetite stimulation within the first few days of administration (Table 5-2); may use calorie counts to gauge its efficacy; moderately anticholinergic; increases digoxin levels; quinidine-like effect; increased QRS, QT, decreased T amplitude, LBBB, 2nd-degree AV block; ventricular arrhythmias as with tricyclics; extrapyramidal side effects; lowers seizure threshold

Resistant Depression: May use nortriptyline in combination w SSRI (Br J Psychiatry 1992;161:562)

PSYCHIATRY

Table 5-2. Antidepressants and Appetite

Antidepressants That Increase Appetite	Antidepressants That Decrease Appetite
Amoxapine	SSRIs
Amitriptyline (sweet craving)*	Imipramine
Doxepin (sweet craving)*	Desipramine
	Trazadone

*Talley JH, Family Practice audiotape, Chapel Hill, NC, 1989.

Enhancers:
- L-Thyroxine 0.025 mg po qd
- Methylphenidate (Ritalin) 0.25–1.00 mg po bid–tid (if alone: 5 mg bid, increase gradually to 10 bid) (Am J Psychiatry 1995; 152:929), or
- Lithium (Nurs Home Pract 1995;3:17) trial for 2 wk (Arch Gen Psychiatry 1994;50:387); up to 300 mg po tid (follow 12-h post-dose levels); obtain levels q 5 d (maximum initial therapeutic dose at trough = 1.2–1.5 mEq/L, then 0.8–1.2 mEq/L to prevent toxicity); in elderly half-life = 36 h; ck TSH, BUN, Cr q 6 mo; withdrawal of caffeine may cause lithium toxicity (Biol Psychiatry 1995;37:348); carbamazepine increases neurotoxicity of lithium: lethargy, ataxia, muscle weakness, tremors, hyperreflexia; *early toxic effects:* early: flu-type aching joints, sniffles, stiffness; *"benign" toxic effects:* nausea, vomiting, diarrhea, polyurea, polydipsia, fine tremor, weight gain, edema; *acute toxicity:* persistent vomiting, uncontrollable diarrhea, hyperactive DTRs, dysarthria, lethargy, somnolence, seizures, coma, and death; *chronic toxicity:* manifested as goitrogenic hypothyroidism, DI, tubular necrosis; lithium can be lowered by urinary alkalinization; if need diuretic, use amiloride instead of thiazide because lithium competes w sodium reabsorption at the proximal tubule; increased lithium levels from <2-gm/d sodium diet, thiazides, NSAIDs, ACE inhibitors
- MAO inhibitors: increase storage of norepinephrine, epinephrine, serotonin; tranylcypromine (Parnate) 10 mg bid and up to 60 mg/d; use tranylcypromine because reversible in 24 h; used for atypical depression as well: hyperphagia, hypersomnia, panic attacks; more safe than tricyclics for heart block, ventricular arrhythmias; most common side effects are sedation, therefore do not give

before 4 pm, and hypotension 3–4 wk into rx course because there is an accumulation of dopamine at the sympathetic ganglion; affects all catecholamine precursors: levodopa, OTC cold remedies, tyramine which increases BP; serotonergic syndrome consists of rigidity, diaphoresis, hyperthermia, coma, and death; meperidine (Demerol) increases serotonin release; MAO-B inhibitors have same effects as MAO-A inhibitors when given at higher doses (30 mg)

Electroshock therapy (Am J Ger Psychiatry 1993;1:30) very effective in the elderly (Nejm 1984;311:163); clear explanation to pt and family because of historical perception of "violence" of rx; don't wait too long (Sci Am 1996;13(8)); *indications:* drug-resistant or intolerant pts, delusional depression, pts w life-threatening behavior (suicidal, catatonic, stuporous); usually 6–8 rx's spaced a day or two apart, 3×/wk more rapid recovery; minimize side effects by placing both stimulus electrodes to nondominant side, brief pulse, minimal duration of stimulus, mortality = 1/10000, relapse rate 10%–20% w maintenance drugs; *contraindications:* absolute: intracranial space-occupying lesion; relative: MI in last 3 mo, severe osteoporosis; <1 mo s/p CVA (J Am Ger Soc 1987;35:516; Convuls Ther 1989;5:75), β-blocker for known ischemic heart disease prevents cardiac complications, should also monitor for arrhythmias, bronchospasm, and signs of aspiration; if delirium occurs early in the course of ECT do w/u; dementia not contraindication to ECT

Depression Associated w Parkinson's: Nortriptyline, desipramine, bupropion, ECT also improve tremor, rigidity, bradykinesia

Psychotic Depression: Antidepressants and antipsychotics or ECT

Mania: Carbamazepine (side effects: rash, sedation, memory problems, decreased wbc), valproate (side effects: gi upset, transient hair loss, tremors); lorazepam, and haloperidol 0.5–1.0 mg qd early to control agitation

Team Management: Short-term group therapy (12 wk) utilizing reminiscent therapy, cognitive therapy, behavioral therapy and limited to small groups (about 6–10 pts) improves self-esteem, insight, social interaction, compliance, and decreases somatization

Model goal setting w family

Music therapy: improvement in depression scores even after 9-mo f/u period (J Gerontol 1994;49:P265)

PSYCHIATRY

Nursing Home: Nurses provide important dx information about nonmajor depression (J Am Ger Soc 1995;43:1118)

Individual therapy or group therapy can help in situations involving caregiver stress

ANXIETY

J Clin Psychiatry 1994;55(suppl):5; Am J Psychiatry 1993;1:46; 1994; 151:640

Cause: Primary anxiety or mood disorders, medical illness/treatment, psychosocial stressors, drug withdrawal

Epidem: Estimates of anxiety prevalence may be falsely low because it may not be admitted by the elderly or adequately recognized by caregivers; DSM-described anxiety disorders less common in elderly, 3.5%–5.5% in those >65 yr old;

Anxiety disorders and phobias (30% of all anxiety states–Small G, Intensive Geriatric Review Center, UCLA, 1/96) most common; agoraphobia is the anxiety disorder with the highest prevalence of onset late in life; new agoraphobia in this age group attributed to exaggerated fears of physical illnesses, falls, or muggings; <11% of agoraphobics have coexisting panic disorder; rate of phobias no different in 65–74-yr olds than those >75 yr old in the community

New-onset panic disorder uncommon in old age (0.3% and virtually all are women and associated w CAD, COPD, gi problems)

Obsessive-compulsive disorder may occur for the first time in old age in women; obsessive-compulsive and panic disorders more likely to persist in old age

Posttraumatic stress disorder 70% early-onset persisting into old age (Am J Psychiatry 1994;2:239)

Parkinsonian pts much higher rates of anxiety than pts w arthritis or MS; anxiety in medical pts much less common in old (2%–13%) than in young (10%–40%)

Pathophys: Serotonin abnormalities resulting in depression, anxiety (J Clin Psychiatry 1994 55:2), medical illnesses (thyroid disease, COPD), or meds/drugs that may induce or exacerbate anxiety (aminophylline, levodopa, prednisone, caffeine, OTC decongestants, alcohol or benzodiazepine withdrawal)

Sx: Tachycardia, tremulousness, flushing, restlessness, unsteadiness, light-headedness, and sleep disturbances; somatic and anxiety-related complaints often mask depression

Si: Hyperventilation, depressed mood

Crs: R/o dysmorphic disorder (fear of going outside because of perceived physical deficit, rx w SSRIs)

Cmplc: Panic disorder: increased mortality, CVD; increased smoking, drug and alcohol abuse

Lab/Xray: TSH, T_4, possibly CBC, lytes, chest xray, and EKG for evidence of organic disease; hx, mental status exam, and physical exam (eg, BP) may suggest further studies such as urine metanephrines or 5HIAA, or head CT (Mayo Clin Proc 1995;70:1999)

Rx: Identify and eliminate stressors when possible; provide support and companionship; instruction in muscle relaxation techniques; possible cognitive psychotherapy; if pharmacotherapy added, always consider risk of side effects vs benefit of treatment; treat depression if present

Trazodone can cause orthostatic hypotension; nefazodone (Serzone) very effective

Tricyclics, eg, nortriptyline and desipramine, are secondary amines with less anticholinergic effects; β-blockers reduce physical sx's but not necessarily emotional sx's; SSRIs have low overdose risk, may either decrease or increase anxiety, insomnia; fluvozaxime (Luvox) approved for obsessive-compulsive disorder symptoms; risperidone, thioridazine (Mellaril) useful as first-line treatment of agitated, anxious pts with dementia or psychosis; antihistamines may induce confusion; buspirone HCl: 6–8-wk trial period may be effective at very low dose 2.5 mg qd to decrease anxiety/agitation in demented pts; lorazepam available im, iv; oxazepam and temazepam rather than those with long-acting breakdown products if possible; wean benzodiazepines slowly over several months to avoid acute withdrawal sx's in the elderly

Team Management: Discover reversible etiologies, behavioral therapies, short-term cognitive therapy (5 sessions), long-term exposure therapy (exposure to anxiety precipitant), observe carefully for benefits or negative effects of rx

SUBSTANCE MISUSE

Cause: Increased need to treat emotional and physical pain, most commonly for arthritis and sleep; increased risk of drug-drug interaction because 4 OTC drugs daily, and if chronically ill, 10–15 drugs daily (women prescribed more than men)

Epidem: 5% of older adults abuse drugs; 80% drug reactions are from minor tranquilizers, sedatives—propoxyphene (Darvon), diazepam (Valium), chlordiazepoxide (Librium)

Pathophys: Reduction of renal and hepatic function; decreased body water and increased fat proportionally; displacement of one drug from protein-binding site by another makes drug-drug interaction more common and complex to treat

Sx: "Doctor shopping," "lost pills," anxiety, amnesia, memory loss, depressed mood, agitation, falls, abdominal pain or constipation, personal hygiene deterioration, confusion, obtundation

Crs: Drug withdrawal longer in older pts; benzodiazepine withdrawal mortality higher

Lab: Drug levels in abuse or w enzyme-competing drugs; LFTs may be elevated

Rx: Treat drug withdrawal in medically monitored setting due to risk of hyperautonomic syndrome, delirium, or convulsion; lipid-soluble benzodiazepines cause more difficult withdrawal (diazepam, chlordiazepoxide); may take months; less lipid-soluble, cut one-half dose for 2 wk, next one-fourth dose for 1 wk, then last one-fourth over 1–2 wk, and monitor vital signs; sedative hypnotic withdrawal 10–21 d; opioids tapered 5–10 d, use alternative pain relief

Team Management: Chemical dependency unit especially important for elderly withdrawal of sedative/hypnotics; consider NA/AA; psychosocial issues need addressing; abuse/misuse may be self-treatment of stresses or losses of late life; pt education of potential for interaction of complex med regimen and its enhanced effect in elderly

ALCOHOL MISUSE

Cause: Reduced tolerance, lower body water for a given amount of alcohol resulting in more pronounced effects; used inappropriately for sleep, pain, loneliness; health professionals may reinforce denial because of unexamined stereotypes, atypical presentation delays diagnosis

Epidem: Prevalence of ETOH abuse is 3% in the community, 10:1 M/F (Jama 1993;270:1222), 18% of general medical inpatients, and 44% of psychiatric inpatients

Pathophys:

- Between ages 25–60, proportion of total body weight that is fat increases by 200% in men, 50% in women; decreased volume of distribution in elderly increases blood ETOH concentration per unit dose of ETOH; moderate drinking in elderly should be defined as no more than 1 drink qd
- Increased permeability of blood-brain barrier leads to greater medical morbidity in the elderly alcoholic
- Two thirds of elderly alcoholics have had lifelong problems with ETOH ("early onset"); one-third develop habits later in life ("late onset")

Sx: Drinking 5–6 d/wk, 4–5 drinks per occasion, confusion (10% of dementias, alcohol-related), self-neglect, CAST/MAST screens have decreased sens in the elderly, more sensitive when also ask about quantity and frequency (Jama 1996;276:1964); self-reported rates of consumption may not accurately indicate impact on elderly lifestyle; tend to be nonspecific: "failure to thrive," insomnia, diarrhea, incontinence, repeated falls, loss of libido, increased metabolism of some drugs (eg, tolbutamide (Orinase), phenytoin (Dilantin)); have high index of suspicion if hospitalized pt develops new-onset seizures, agitation, confusion, anxiety, medical rx not working

Si: In general, increased lab abnormalities; high MCV, abnormal LFTs, multiple spider nevi

Crs: Improved prognosis w late age of onset of alcoholism, social and family support, absence of dementia; drug withdrawal can take longer

Cmplc: Watch for ETOH-med interactions, especially CNS depressants: benzodiazepines, barbiturates, diphenhydramine (Benadryl), psychotropics; ETOH interacts with 50% of most prescribed meds!; can precipitate hypoglycemic episodes in IDDM

Rx:

Prevention: Pt education to help elderly understand that habitual use of alcohol as aging advances may interfere with achievement of optimal health and functioning in context of increasing chronic disease conditions; avoid trap that the pt has only a few years left, so why not enjoy?; emphasize effect of alcohol on sleep pattern, nutrition, energy

Therapeutic (Clin Ger Med 1993;9:197; Prim Care 1993;20:155):
- Treat withdrawal w thiamine, Mg if <1 mEq/L w 0.25–0.50 mEq/kg/d, one-third to one-half average adult benzodiazepine dose reducing by 10%/d; long-acting benzodiazepine may be better for withdrawing from high-milligram-potency benzodiazepines; ensure hydration; detoxification may take months, postpone w/u of cognitive loss several weeks; do not prescribe disulfiram (Antabuse) because elderly susceptible to disulfiram reaction w resultant cardiac complications
- Watch for reactive depression and treat with SSRI

Team Management:
- Rehab units 1–3 wk; AA (about one-third AA participants >50 yr old), or social situations that help elderly pursue an abstinent lifestyle
- Involve pt's pharmacy to monitor prescription refills, outreach program
- Patient education: alcohol affects medical conditions, precipitating hypoglycemic reactions in IDDM, interacts w 50% of most prescribed drugs
- Explore family constellation: chief enabler, family hero, scapegoat, lost child, mascot

DEMENTIAS

See Table 5-3 on pp. 114–115.

CORTICAL DEMENTIA (DEMENTIA, ALZHEIMER'S TYPE (DAT))

Ann IM 1991;115:122; Nejm 1986;314:964; Clin Ger Med 1994;10: 239; Med Clin N Am 1994;78:811; Sultzer DL, Cummings JL, Intensive Geriatric Review Course, UCLA, 1/96; Nejm 1996;335:330; Sci Amer 1997;11:xi

Cause: 20%–40% genetic transmission, autosomal dominant, chromosome 12 (Jama 1997;277:775); family hx imparts 3–4× risk of general population; head trauma imparts 3× risk of general population; most are acquired and of unclear etiology; toxins eg carbon dioxide, carbon monoxide; elevated risk of subsequent strokes in older persons w cognitive impairment suggesting CVD plays important role in causing cognitive impairment (J Am Ger Soc 1996;44: 237); low linguistic ability in early life strong predictor of poor cognitive function and Alzheimer's in late life (Jama 1996;275: 582)

Epidem: Prevalence = 5% at age 70, 20% at 80, 50% at 90 (Jama 1995;273:1354); 20% incidence in family members of late-onset Alzheimer's pts (Ann IM 1991;115:601); males = females; 100% of Down syndrome pts age >35 yr (Science 1992;258:668; Ann IM 1985;103:526); nondemented elderly w depressed mood more at risk for developing Alzheimer's dementia (Arch Gen Psychiatry 1996;53:175)

40+% of elderly dementia is purely Alzheimer's, the rest is vascular multi-infarct type predominantly (Nejm 1993;328:153); 70% of NH pts have Alzheimer's dementia; "mixed dementia" felt to be common

Associated w E4 allele of apolipoprotein E (Jama 1995;273:1274) which facilitates β-amyloid protein deposition in neurofibrillary tangles (Nejm 1995;333:1242); E2 allele protective against the development of Alzheimer's (Jama 1996;275:1612)

Higher antioxidants: ascorbic acid and β-carotene plasma levels are associated w better memory performance (Jags 1997; 45:718)

Pathophys: Structural changes most severe in hippocampus and association cortex of parietal, temporal, frontal lobes; atrophy of corpus callosum differentiates Alzheimer's from healthy elderly and incipient dementia (J Am Ger Soc 1996;44:798); neurofibrillary tangles are paired helical filaments that contain tau and ubiquitin proteins associated w intracellular microtubules (Nejm 1991;325:1849);

Table 5-3. Dementias

	Delerium—Infecting, Metabolic, etc.	AD (60%)	Frontal Lobe Dementia (10%), Pick's (1–2%)	Subcortical (2–3%) (Huntington's, Wilson's, SNP, NPH, Parkinson's)	Vascular Dementias (15%) (Multi-infarct, Binswanger's Cortical Infarctions)	Wernicke-Korsakoff
History Onset, duration	Sudden, hours-days (CJD-dementia die within 1 yr)	Insidious, month–years; 8–10 yr AD	2–10 yr	—	Acute, stepwise[a]	—
Mental status Attention	Fluctuating[a]	—	—	—	—	—
Memory Learning, recall, and recognition	Impaired by poor attention	Amnesia early	Amnesia late[a]	Forgetful[a] (retrieval deficit)	—	—
Language Comprehension, repetition, naming	Normal or mild anomia, misnaming, dysgraphia, may be impaired	Aphasia	—	Normal[a]	—	—
Speech	Slurred	Normal	Stereotyped speech, terminal mutism	Abnormal (hypophonic, dysarthric, mute)	—	—
Perception Visual spatial skills, constructional apraxia	Hallucination	Visual spatial	Visual spatial disturbance late	Impaired	—	—
Cognition Calculation, abstraction, judgment	—	Abnormal[a] (acalculia, poor judgment, impaired abstraction)	Calculations spared early	Abnormal (slowed, dilapidated)	—	Confabulation early, antegrade memory loss[a]; can't learn new things

Executive skills Drive, programming response control synthesis	Very poor	—	Impairment of initiation, goal setting, planning	Problems with executive skills	—	—
Mood affect	Fear, suspiciousness may often be prominent	Paranoid delusions, 25% disinterested or uninhibited	Personality change early,[a] Klüver-Bucy[b] syndrome, apathy, irritability, jocularity, euphoria, loss of fear	Abnormal (apathetic or depressed), blunting, emotional withdrawal	Preservation of personality; emotional lability	Placid, congenial
Motor Posture, tone, movement, gait	Postural tremor, myoclonus, asterixis; AIDS: psychomotor slowing, focal neurologic signs	Normal into final stages (then increased tone and flexed posture)	—	Posture-stooped,[a] SNP (extended or flexed) (Parkinson's) tone, increased, tremor, bradykinesia, chorea, dystonia, abnormal gait	Multifocal defects in lacunar disease, rigid, EPS, pseudobulbar palsy	Nystagmus, ataxia (detectable in late stages)

AD = Alzheimer's; SNP = supranuclear palsy, CJC = Creutzfeldt-Jakob disease; AIDS = acquired immunodeficiency syndrome; SNP = supranuclear palsy; EPS = extrapyramidal syndromes.

[a] Most characteristic findings.

[b] Klüver-Bucy—blunted emotional response, hypersex, gluttony.

Modified from tables in Cummings, Benson, and Loverme, 1980; Sultzer/Cummings intensive course in geriatric medicine, 1/96.

neuronal dropout; decreased acetylcholine synthesis (Nejm 1985; 313:7), hence anticholinergics worsen (Nejm 1985;313:7); amyloid A4 protein deposition perhaps (Lancet 1992;340:467; Ann Neurol 1992;32:157); gene located on chomosomes 14, 19, 21 (Nejm 1989;320:1446); whether plaques are a consequence of altered metabolism or are primary causative lesions—area of active debate (Neuron 1996;16:921)

Sx: Loss of social skills and memory usually unacknowledged by pt unless early stages; depression related to insight into cognitive losses

Si: Abnormal mental status (Psychiatr Clin N Am 1991;14:309) w memory loss >6 mo + ≥2 other cognitive function impairments for definition of dementia according to National Institute of Neurological and Communicative Disorders and Stroke–Alzheimer's Disease and Related Disorders (NINCDS-ADRDA); these criteria produce 90%–100% accuracy (Neurol 1993;43:250); DSM IV only requires one cognitive deficit for definition of dementia, producing 80%–85% accuracy (American Psychiatric Association, DSM IV, 1994:142); proper interpretation of Mini Mental State Exam (MMSE) requires knowledge of pt's reading level (J Am Ger Soc 1995;43:807)

Family key to earliest dx if can be encouraged to share information; spousal denial and covering of sx of losses common; retrospective imaging suggests 3–4 yr of sx's before presentation to health professional

- Memory, recent much worse than remote; including orientation to time (d, mo, yr) (day of week is 53% sens, 92% specif) (Ann IM 1991;115:122); recall 3 items (medial temporal lobe-hippocampus, mammillary bodies, hypothalamus)
- Perceptive/spatial disorientation, eg, answers to "How do you get there from here?"; clock face drawing; copy interlocking pentagons (parietal, frontal, occipital)
- Language impairments: anomias/paraphasias/aphasias which often result in neologisms or circumlocutions, fluent aphasia (posterior L brain–Wernicke); use of automatic phrases and cliches; as pt progresses, ask questions that only require short answers to demonstrate comprehension: "Point to the light," "Do you put your shoes on before your socks?" "Is my wife's brother a man

or a woman?" "The lion was killed by the tiger. Which animal is dead?"

- Scoring: <21 on the MMSE is abnormal for 8th-grade education, <23 is abnormal for high school education, <24 abnormal for college education, 18–24 mild cognitive impairment, 0–17 severe cognitive impairment; MMSE insensitive to noncortical dementias, Hachinski scale helps discriminate other dementias from Alzheimer's dementia
- Abstraction impairments: "What does it mean to give someone the cold shoulder?", categorization, calculations
- Executive skills: motivation, ability to initiate activity, ability to recognize patterns, generate motor programs, and the ability to plan and execute a strategy, alternate square and triangle pattern (frontal lobe) (Exp Aging Res 1994;20:73); highly correlated w the appearance of problem behaviors in Alzheimer's dementia (Exp Aging Res 1994;20:73)
- Affect changes and poor judgment: neuropsychiatric findings with other assessment tests (J Fam Pract 1993;37:599)
- Impairment of verbal memory and category naming associated w incipient dementia (Neurol 1995;45:957)
- Pupillary dilatation >20% within 30 min to 1/100 diluted tropicamide gtts, present very early even 1 yr before measurable DAT, 95% sens and specif (Sci 1994;266:1051); controversial—no change in dilatation noted (Arch Neurol 1997;54:55)

Crs: Slowly progressive; mean survival from first sx = 10 yr, shorter the more severe it is (Ann IM 1990;113:429); average decline per year = 3 points on the MMSE, poor prognosis w extrapyramidal signs or psychosis (Jama 1997;277:806); stages (Am J Psychiatry 1982, 139:1136) 1 and 2, forget familiar names and places; stage 3, family and coworkers aware; stage 4, difficulty w finances; stage 5, need assistance dressing; stage 6, incontinence, delusional; stage 7, grunting, nonambulatory

Personality changes (from progressive passivity to marked hostility) can develop before cognitive impairments (J Ger Psychiatry Neurol 1990;3:21)

Delusions of paranoid type most common, accusations of theft, infidelity; hallucinations usually visual in 25% of pts

Depression in 40%

Lewy body variant: intraneural inclusion bodies on histopathology, cortical-type cognitive impairment, extrapyramidal signs (Neurol 1990;40:1)

Clinical characteristics of atypical dementia syndromes (Nejm 1996; 335:330), those w language, constructional apraxia out of proportion to memory loss progress less rapidly

Agitated behavior occurs sometime during course of disease in one-third to one-half of pts w Alzheimer's

Cmplc:

R/o (Ann IM 1984;100:417) Reversible Causes (Nejm 1986;314: 1111):

- Delirium, if acute, in which attention span is most prominent deficit; test by serial 7's; serial digits up to 7, eg, phone numbers; spell "world" or do days of week backward; associated w increased mortality (J Am Ger Soc 1992;40:759; Jama 1990;263: 1097); if decline on MMSE is >3–4pts/yr or score of 15 after only 3 yr h/o dementia, must r/o other problems (Folstein M, Bar Harbor, ME, 10/96)

- Independent risk factors for developing delirium in hospital include preexisting dementia, >80 yr old, fracture on admission, symptomatic infection, male gender, use of antipsychotic or narcotic med; septic encephalopathy (Jama 1996;275:470): severity of Glasgow Coma Score correlates w BUN, bilirubin, bacteremia

- Hypothyroidism (depression, irritability, mental slowing); myxedema (4%), thyrotoxicosis less common, psychomotor retardation, apathy, less anxiety, tremor, tachycardia that is characteristic of younger pts; both hypothyroidism and hyperthyroidism can present w frank psychosis

- Drugs, single or multiple drugs (6%)

- Toxins like occult solvent/paint exposure may cause peripheral neuropathy, myopathy, cerebellar signs; elevated blood or urine levels of Pb, As, Hg, manganese, thallium

- Subdural hematoma (2%), results from cerebral atrophy and shearing of already stretched bridging veins during trauma

- Focal neurologic signs common and mistaken for vascular dementia:
  Frontal/temporal tumor
  AIDS: psychomotor slowing, focal neurologic signs, frontal lobe cell loss

Jakob-Creutzfeldt, rare, slow virus, incubation period several
years, no known cure, progresses rapidly, death within a year,
cerebellar and extrapyramidal signs, startle myoclonus, asymmetric slowing or periodic polyspike discharges on EEG

Syphilitic dementia: meningovascular (2–10 yr, sometimes 30–40
yr after initial infection); inflammatory arteritis that can result
in stroke and vascular dementia; general paresis (7–12 yr
after initial infection); delusions, hallucinations, mood disorders often present; pseudobulbar palsy; poor coordination;
hyperreflexia or hyporeflexia; pupillary abnormalities; signs of
posterior column dysfunction (taboparesis); VDRL and rapid
plasma reagent nonreactive in one-fourth of pts w late neurosyphilis; fluorescent treponema antibody (FTA) more sensitive
but remains positive even after treatment

Vit B_{12} deficiency: irritability, psychosis, delirium, amnesia, slowing of thought processes may also occur; peripheral neuropathy, optic atrophy, older pts symptomatic at higher levels of
vit B_{12} (low nl) than younger pts (J Am Ger Soc 1996;44:
1355)

Depression pseudodementia: more "I don't know" answers than
the "guesses" of DAT; lack of progression of sx's; preserved
awareness of deficits; preserved language skills; cued recall nl;
impaired problem solving and word list generation; also often
both (depression and dementia) occur together

Wernicke-Korsakoff syndrome w anterograde memory loss, alcohol hx; may recover partially over 1 yr (Nejm 1985;312:16)

R/o (Ann IM 1984;100:417) Nonreversible Causes:
• Age-associated memory impairment (AAMI), also termed *benign*,
and if more severe, *malignant senescent forgetfulness*, may be an
early monosymptomatic stage of Alzheimer's dementia; lower *N*-
acetyl-acetate in AAMI and DAT brains than in normal aging
brain (J Am Ger Soc 1996;44:133)
• Age-associated cognitive decline (AACD), a transitional state
between normal aging but does not meet criteria for global cognitive deficit of dementia; no memory impairment
• Subcortical dementias which show forgetfulness, executive dysfunction (J Am Ger Soc 1997;45:386), and motor findings early
(Arch Neurol 1993;50:873), unlike the amnesia and early language deficits in DAT: eg, Parkinson's (slowing of cognition),

less agnosia than w cortical dementias and more apathy than w cortical dementias; diffuse Lewy body disease (DLBD) (hallucinations occur earlier than, and extrapyramidal dysfunction more mild than w Parkinson's–Neurol 1994;35:81); progressive supranuclear palsy (axial rigidity, vertical gaze palsy, may respond to amitriptyline 10–40 mg bid–J Am Ger Soc 1996;44:1072); spinocerebellar degenerations, Huntington's, Wilson's, olivopontine degeneration, and NPH (obstruction of CSF flow around the convexity of the brain, impaired absorption into the sagittal sinus, gait abnormalities initial symptom w small shuffling steps w feet set down at variable force, postural instability, difficulties w fine hand movements, lack of initiative and slowness of thought, best outcomes of shunt done earlier in disease, may be partially reversible, not without substantial morbidity, see p 132); systemic diseases: end-stage renal failure, CHF, COPD, DM (subcortical microvascular lesions and hippocampal damage from hypoglycemia)

- Multi-infarct dementia: stepwise crs, emotional lability prominent, and h/o HT, CVA, or ASHD; features of mixed cortical/subcortical dementia, see vascular dementias, p 132)
- Alcohol-related dementias: 10–15-yr drinking hx, apathy and noncortical features predominate, irritability, may have nl MMSE, partially reversible w abstinence, direct toxic effect of alcohol has not been established
- Pick's disease (1%–2% cases, argentophilic inclusion bodies or Pick body on histopathology), if no histopathology—then frontal-temporal dementia (J Am Ger Soc 1997;45:579) similar to Alzheimer's but much younger onset with less memory impairment and more behavioral change (apathy, irritability, jocularity, euphoria, *Klüver-Bucey syndrome* = emotional blunting, loss of fear, oral exploratory behavior, change in eating habits, altered sexual activity), disordered executive function (impairment of initiation goal setting planning); 2–10-yr duration; no praxis or visuospatial deficit as w Alzheimer's; language-abundant unfocused speech, echolalia, palilalia; is rare and anatomic changes are isolated to frontal and temporal lobes; other frontal lobe dementias comprise 10% of dementias (frontal lobe degeneration

of the non-Alzheimer's type, progressive subcortical gliosis, amyotrophic lateral sclerosis (ALS)–dementia syndrome); MMSE may be nl w early frontal lobe, Lewy body, Pick's dementias

- Paraphrenia: hallucinations and delusions out of proportion to intellectual dysfunction

Lab: Cost-effectiveness of w/u for reversible dementias questionable (J Neurol 1995;242:446); guidelines for evaluation from Agency for Health Care Policy and Research (Neurol 1995;45:211)

Pathology: Brain histology at postmortem shows neurofibrillary tangles, senile plaques with eosinophilic amyloid

Hematology: CBC

Chemistry: T_3, T_4, chem panel, lytes if acute, vit B_{12} level, folate, UA

Serology: VDRL, perhaps HIV antibody if young, dementia occurs in 20% HIV pts

Noninvasive: EEG occasionally helpful to distinguish DAT (slow waves) from depression (nl); toxic, metabolic, or partial complex seizure or Jakob-Creutzfeldt

Obtain CSF in subacute cases

APOE (genotyping for E allele) positive predictive value very high but negative predictive value nil

Xray: Chest xray (NIH Consensus Development Conference Statement 1987;6(11)); head CT or MRI distinguishes from multi-infarct dementia—periventricular hyperintensities on T2-weighted images w multi-infarct dementia and in deep white matter w Alzheimer's (Neurol 1993;43:250); only if si's of subdural or rapid onset (Ann IM 1984;100:417); in all possibly? (Nejm 1986;314:964); very low yield of reversible disease, eg, <1/250; CT, MRI not helpful unless focal findings present (Ann IM 1994;120:856)

If motor dysfunction, eg, rigidity, reflex asymmetry, abnormal reflexes, then obtain MRI to detect stroke and ischemic changes (J Am Ger Soc 1995;43:138); MRI better than CT for subcortical pathology

PET, SPECT: Decreased cerebral blood flow and glucose metabolism in parietal, temporal, frontal association cortex bilaterally (Arch Neurol 1995;52:773); mostly a research tool at this point; as early treatment evolves these will become more clinically applicable tests; low sens and specif of SPECT in Alzheimer's (J Am Ger Soc 1997;45:15)

PSYCHIATRY

Rx:

Preventive: Apolipoprotein E screening not appropriate (Jama 1997;277:832)

Therapeutic:

- Memory aids (J Fam Pract 1993;37:6)
- Acetylcholine esterase inhibitors like physostigmine and tacrine (tetrahydroaminoacridine (THA, Cognex) (Jama 1994;271:985; Med Let Drugs Ther 1993;35:87; Am Fam Phys 1994;50:819), 10 mg qid (check serum ALT q wk × 6 wk), increase by 10 mg q 6 wk, maximum dose = 40 mg qid × several months to see effect, may help cognition but in a clinically insignificant way (Jama 1992;268:2523); 30% of pts respond w improvement of MMSE score of about 1–2 points (Nejm 1992;327:1253,1306); favorable effect on noncognitive symptoms such as delusions (Nejm 1990;322:1272; 1991;323:349), may also help w Lewy body dementia (Nurs Home Med 1995;3:300); more likely to have clinically relevant response to tacrine if mild to moderate dementia, w relative preservation of language and praxis

    Adverse effects: 25% of pts have to be withdrawn from tacrine because of liver enzyme elevation; permanent hepatic damage in 21%; 10%–20% gi distress that results in discontinuation of med; tacrine combined w neuroleptic can cause Parkinson's (J Clin Psychopharmacol 1995;15:284); donepezil (Aricept) 5 mg po (Med Let 1997;39:53; J Clin Psychiatry 1996;57:30), which may be increased to 10 mg after 6 wk, like tacrine has similar MMSE improvement, does not affect liver function but has gi side effects, eg, nausea, vomiting, diarrhea, avoid if hx PND, sick sinus syndrome, pulmonary disease, bladder outflow problems (Portney R. Mass General Hospital, presented Waterville, ME Mar '97)

- Doubtfully vasodilators like ergoloid mesylates (Hydergine) 2 mg tid × 6 mo (Ann IM 1984;100:896); no value (Nejm 1990;323:445)

- New drug therapies being developed: pharmacologic interventions against the amyloid cascade, neuroprotective agents such as glutamate antagonists, antioxidants; huperzine A (a compound first isolated from traditional Chinese herbal medicine), potent inhibitor acetylcholinesterase, may also protect neurons (Jama

Table 5-4. Medications for Agitated Demented Patients

Insomnia, Anxiety, Fear, Tension	Depressed Mood, Crying	Hostile, Assaultive, Psychotic
Benzodiazepine, oxazepam up to 10 mg qid, or propranolol up to 40 qid plus buspirone	Antidepressant, trazodone 25 mg up to 200 mg/d or SSRIs	Carbamazepine 25 tid up to 400 mg/d (level = 7), or risperidone 0.5 mg or antipsychotic (see Table 5-5)

Adapted from Arch IM 1995;155:250.

1997;277:276) injection of neurotrophic agents into ventricular system to retard neural degeneration (Nurs Home Med 1995;3:3E)
- Estrogen protective (Horm Metab Res 1995;27:204; J Am Ger Soc 1996;44:865); NSAIDs protective (J Am Ger Soc 1996;44:1025,1307)
- Vit E and monoamine oxidose-B inhibitors eg selegiline 5 g po bid may have neurotropic effects as well (Nejm 1997;336:1216,1245; Science 1997;276:675)
- Of agitated behavior (Table 5-4)

Antipsychotic drug uses: antiaggressive effects of antipsychotics may take up to 8 wk to appear, pts w severe dementia do not respond as well; agitation may result from benzodiazepine withdrawal (Am J Hosp Pharm 1994;51:2917)

Government-approved indications for antipsychotic drug use in NH: biting, kicking, scratching, or other aggressive behaviors presenting as danger to self or others; functional impairment caused by continuous crying out, screaming, pacing, hallucinations, paranoia, or delusions; documentation of frequency and duration (Omnibus Nursing Home required, Fed Reg 1992;57:4519)

Phenothiazines, in order of increasing extrapyramidal and decreasing sedation/anticholinergic/hypotensive effects (Table 5-5): Mellaril (thioridazine), Thorazine (chlorpromazine), Navane (thiothixene), Haldol (halperidol), Prolixin (fluphenazine)—mnemonic = "My troubles now have passed"; one-fifth to one-fourth dose used in younger person

Extrapyramidal side effects: acute dystonic reactions rare in the elderly (Consult Pharm 1992;7:921), treated w diphenhydramine (Benadryl); parkinsonian signs treated w benztropine mesylate

PSYCHIATRY

Table 5-5. Antipsychotic Drugs

Antipsychotic	Side Effect Profile	
	Hypotension, Sedation, Anticholinergic	**EPS**
Mellaril ("my")	+++++	+
Thorazine ("troubles")	++++	++
Navane ("now")	+++	+++
Haldol ("have")	++	++++
Prolixin ("passed")	+	+++++

EPS = extrapyramidal syndrome.

(Cogentin) or anticholinergic or amantadine for 3 mo, or switching to lower-potency antipsychotic; akathisia: 20% prevalence, anticholinergics not as effective at treating as benzodiazepines, or β-blockers for effects on GABA (Am J Hosp Pharm 1991;48:1271); also w amantadine, diazepam (Valium), tardive dyskinesia: prevalence as high as 40% and more severe w age (J Am Ger Soc 1987;35:233), $2\times$ more frequent in blacks than whites, increasing antipsychotic dose when this sx first appears will eliminate it temporarily (supersensitization of dopaminergic receptors after prolonged receptor blockade, abnormal movements can paradoxically worsen when the dosage of the antipsychotic is first decreased), anticholinergics often exacerbate it, greatest risk first 2 yr of treatment (Small, Intensive Geriatric Review Course, UCLA, 1996); adding lithium to antipsychotic may lead to neuroleptic malignant syndrome (NMS) (J Clin Psychopharmacol; 5–40% tardive dyskinesia eventually remit, can rx w carbamazepine, dopaminergic, and GA-BA-ergic drugs (Valproic acid and Depakene) 1993;54:35)
Orthostatic hypotension: blockade of α_1-receptors more common w low-potency antipsychotics, aliphatic phenothiazines, and clozapine; weight gain
- Clozapine (J Ger Psychiatry Neurol 1994;7:129; Med Let Drugs Ther 1994;36:33; Drug Topics 1994;138:30): avoid extrapyramidal sx (Am J Hlth Syst Pharm 1995;52:S9); no tardive dyskinesia, but causes agranulocytosis in 1%–2% pts, which can be fatal; therefore weekly monitoring and report to national registry

(Med Let Drugs Ther 1993;35:16); older pts at greater risk for leukopenia (Am J Ger Psychiatry 1995;3:26), hypotension, and seizures (J Ger Psychiatry Neurol 1994;7:129) can continue med and rx seizures w valproate (Neurol 1994;44:2247); average dose 37 mg/d (Neurol 1995;45:432); optimal duration of clozapine trial 6 wk–12 mo (Can J Psychiatry 1995;40:208)

Clozapine significantly reduces gastric acid secretion, resulting in decrease in gastric ulcers (Am J Psychiatry 1995;152:821)

Clozapine overdose: mental status changes (somnolence), tachycardia, aspiration pneumonia, hypotension, seizures; no cases of agranulocytosis reported with overdose; death rare (J Emerg Med 1995;13:199)

Drug interactions: clozapine and tricyclic antidepressant may produce delirium due to additive anticholinergic effects; cimetidine induced toxicity because of inhibition of cytochrome P-450

Kinetics: cleared mostly through hepatic enzyme metabolism; start w 6.25 mg to avoid bradycardia (J Clin Psychiatry 1995; 56:180)

- Risperidone: decreases neg (depression, social withdrawal, apathy) as well as pos sx's (delusions, hallucinations, paranoia, sx of schizophrenia); diminishes depression through its antagonism of 5-HT$_2$ receptors (American Medical Directors Association 19th annual symposium, New Orleans, LA, 3/7/96); also better than other phenothiazines for Lewy dody dementia (Nurs Home Med 1995;3:300); not anticholinergic; rarely causes sedation at low doses; starting dose 0.5 mg qd or bid w slow titration avoids hypotension (J Ger Psychiatry Neurol 1995;8:159), little in the way of drug interactions; when tapering clozapine and beginning risperidone, watch clozapine levels carefully (Psychiatr Drug Alerts 1996;2:9); extrapyramidal side effects dose-dependent (>10 mg/d); no tardive dyskinesia or agranulocytosis reported; may see elevation of prolactin, weight gain, sexual dysfunction

Kinetics: well absorbed from gi tract; unaffected by food; more rapid onset of action than clozapine, producing clinical response after 1 wk; extensively metabolized by the liver, excreted in urine, partly in feces; elimination half-life – 20 h; available in 1-, 2-, 3-, 4-mg tabs; cost comparison: haloperidol (Haldol) = $21–$79, risperidone = $237, clozapine = $308

- Olanzapine: serotonin-dopamine antagonist w little extrapyramidal side effects, but side effect profile otherwise very much like clozapine, 5–20 mg qd (30 hr half-life), 2.5 mg in NH pts (NH Med 1997;5:supplement 7F)
- Mood stabilizers/anticonvulsants: carbamazepine effective in treatment of agitation, aggressiveness, impulsivity, and sexually inappropriate behaviors; 25 mg po bid up to 200 tid to a level of 6–7 mg/dL, following CBC and LFTs (J Clin Psychiatry 1990; 51:115); valproic acid may reduce aggression, temper outbursts, and agitation (J Neuropsychiatry Clin Neurosci 1995;7:314); ASA may increase valproic acid levels, can cause diarrhea
- Benzodiazepines for anxiety but not for chronic use: eg, oxazepam (Serax) 10 mg po tid, or lorazepam (Ativan) 0.5–1.0 mg qid, but diminished effect after several months; agitation can be a result of benzodiazepine withdrawal; clonazepam stimulates serotonin production and may lessen aggressive behavior, hyperactivity, social intrusiveness, and impulsivity
- Azaperone when given w neuroleptic drugs decreases severity of tardive dyskinesia, improves akathisia and parkinsonism, eg, buspirone 60 mg/d (Buspar) (Phys Postgrad Press 1994;12:3); switching from benzodiazepine to azaperone: change short- or intermediate-acting benzodiazepine (eg, alprazolam (Xanax)) to long-acting (eg, clonazepam (Klonopin)), add azaperone 5–10 mg 3× a day up to 30 mg/d, schedule taper of benzodiazepine over 60–90 d; takes 2–3 wk for azaperone to take effect (Am Fam Phys 1996;53:2349)
- Trazodone is beneficial in treatment of sleep deprivation, aggression, and hostility (J Clin Psychiatry 1995;56:374), give hs because of hypotension
- Propranolol 40–120 mg (Med Clin N Am 1994;78:814)
- Estrogen 1.25 mg qd for sexual aggression in elderly men (J Am Ger Soc 1991;31:1110), medroxyprogesterone (J Clin Psychiatry 1987;48:368); ethics of treatment (Am J Psychiatry 1981;138:5)

Team Management (Tables 5-6, 5-7):
- Meeting w the family (Am Fam Phys 1984;29:149): *first session* (important that pt be included in initial family meeting, may not remember content but will remember being included and taken seriously)

Encourage catharsis re family's burden to explain or cover up Alzheimer secret, the family's loss of social roles and identities; violence from pt's catastrophic reactions, being accused of malevolent motives by the pt, guilt regarding reflex anger to physical abuse by pt, blaming themselves for pt's irritability and withdrawal, difficulties w having to constantly supervise pt

Facilitate learning of family re differences between memory loss and attention deficit; stages of dementia; compliment family and pt for recognizing the problem and dispel myths (pt not lazy, crazy, dementia is not caused by stress, vit deficiency, and not amenable to drill, pts can still feel embarrassment and shame)

Send letters to family members who are geographically separated, who may not have recognized subtle changes in the pt, and who may think the primary care giver is exaggerating the problem

Have family read Alzheimer material and return for a f/u *second session* without the pt: identify where guilt has led to self-sacrificing caregiver behaviors, acknowledge their fears for the future and support them in decisions they must make that may be unacceptable to their afflicted parent or spouse, eg, NH placement (explore cultural values, and family conflicts)

Help family draw up a day-to-day care plan for the pt that will provide a predictable environment and repeated reassurance; learn from family as much as possible about the successful approaches and accomplishments to this stage of disease; acknowledge importance of individualized approach for the pt (spouse) and assure that care plan will integrate their prior work; create a "team" w family and health professionals; emphasize family's important continuing role

Encourage family to participate in support group, continue to meet their own individual needs; reinforce that they are developing expertise that is of value to the community at large, encourage political advocacy when it is voiced by the family

• Behavioral management: look for precipitants of difficult behavior (what, where, why, when, who); reassurance and redirection effective, do not "reality orient" pts w cortical dementia, may result in "catastrophic reaction"; however reality orientation and prompting very important techniques in subcortical dementias;

Table 5-6. C-ADAT: Caregiver's Alzheimer's Disease Assessment Tool

Group	MMSE Mean (±SD)	Characteristic Function and Cognitive Deficit	Approximate Age Function Acquired	Characteristic Function Preserved	Adjuvant Psychological Features	Major Treatment Concerns	Prognosis During 4-yr Follow-up
Forgetfulness (Stage I)	29.6 (±0.7)	None	—	All	None	—	—
Forgetfulness (Stage II)	28.9 (±1.3)	Subjective c/o word finding, forgetting familiar names, normal performance at work	Adult	No objective Memory deficit on clinical interview	Anxiety	Reassurance Treat anxiety	Most will not develop AD but only mild forgetfulness Predicted life expectancy in AD is 8–10 yr
Confusion Stage III	24.6 (±3.5)	Disorientation to time. Clear-cut memory and cognitive deficit Withdrawal from challenging situations (work) Word and name finding deficit	Young adult	Normal ADL and IADL Routine activity well preserved Driving to familiar area	Anxiety Depression	Prevent conditions that increase anxiety Treat depression	80% deterioration in cognitive function Predicted life expectancy 6–8 yr
Dementia Stage IV	20.0 (±3.8)	Disorientation to place Decreased ability to handle finances, perform complex tasks, and remember recent events Decreased driving ability: gets lost, unable to interpret signs	8 yr	Might be oriented ×2 Able to drive to familiar places Able to stay in the community	Denial Paranoid thoughts	Strategy to approach patient with denial Handling finances Use of a notebook as a memory aid Control driving location	25% in nursing home 25% remain in the community Predicted life expectancy 4–6 yr

	MMSE						
Dementia Stage V	14.3 (±3.4)	Require assistance choosing attire Forget to bathe Not able to stay in community without assistance	5–7 yr	Able to dress Able to bathe alone	Agitation Reversed sleep patterns	Full home assistance Day care Prepare for long-term care facility	Most in nursing homes Persistent gradual deterioration Predicted life expectancy 3–4 yr
Dementia Stage VI	8.3 (±4.8)	Not remembering names of spouse, child Require assistance bathing Require assistance dressing Require assistance toileting Urinary incontinent Fecal incontinent	5 yr 4 yr 3 yr 2 yr	Language impaired Walk with small steps	Violent psychosis, eg, hallucination	24-hr home help Nursing home Treatment for agitation and psychosis	Most will die or be in a nursing home
Dementia Stage VII	0 (±0)	Dramatic deterioration in: Speech activity Ambulation Sitting Smile Body posture/head Neurologic cortical signs	15 mo 12 mo 8 mo 4 mo 2 mo	None	None	Soft food diet Nasogastric tube or PEG tube	14% will die from unknown etiology Possible due to defect in the regulation of vital signs, eg, respiratory function

MMSE = Mini-Mental State Exam; c/o = complains of; PEG = percutaneous endoscopic gastrostomy; AD = Alzheimer's.
From Am J Alzheimer Dis Rel Disord Res 1995;10:4.

Table 5-7. Behavior of Demented Patients During Late Stages (Usually in Nursing Home Setting)

Stage V/VII:

Usually placed in NH; aware of surroundings but not aware of their purpose; "all dressed up with nowhere to go"; very unhappy when have to ineract w unkempt, aggressive patients; eg, stage VII/VII patients; enjoy opportunity to look after needy cooperative patients (stage VI/VII)

STATE VI/VII:

Not sure where or who they are; need constant reassurance; "Velcro stage"; get along well w stage V/VII patients; like being led around by them; don't mind stage VII/VII patients; not aware enough to be bothered by them

Stage VII/VII:

If still ambulatory, will follow retreating stimuli; they stop following people when others have stopped moving; tend to follow visitors out of the door of the NH, but are easily redirected

---

From lecture by Lucero M, Lewiston, ME, 1994.

otherwise pts may become depressed when cargivers assume pts are less capable than they are

Hallucinations, delusions = poor prognosis (J Am Ger Soc 1992; 40:768): pts may often conceal so ask subtly: "How are you getting on with other relatives? Neighbors? Are they annoying in any way? Are they deliberately trying to annoy you? Often when one is elderly, other people are unsympathetic—is that a problem?"

Sundowning (increased confusion and agitation in the late afternoon secondary to disturbances in circadian rhythm and REM sleep, deterioration of suprachiasmic nucleus of hypothalamus): restrict daytime sleep, expose to bright light during the day, low-stress activity schedules (J Psychol Nurs 1996; 34:40; Acta Psychiatr Scand 1994;89:1)

Wandering: "goal-directed" (disguise exit signs, place stop signs), "aimless wandering" (provide more structure, investigate possible discomfort)

Repetitive speech: group singing, reminiscing activities

Resistance to care: "Good cop, bad cop" intervention in which
pt is rescued from purposely overbearing caregiver by gentler
caregiver so that the pt will follow the second caregiver and
perform a task they usually resist

Caregivers should be encouraged to recognize their own stress;
"36-h day" day care center

In *NH*, wandering can also be managed by "wandering areas,"
sign posts, pictures of residents on resident room doors, tape
barriers on floors and across doors, half-doors, coded locks

Screaming: hearing augmentation devices for screaming pts to
prevent them from screaming as loud, controversial (Nurs
Hom Med 1997;4:515)

- Driving: score on MMSE and visual tracking can be used to strat-
ify which cognitively impaired pts can drive safely (Clin Ger
Med 1993;9:279; Jama 1995;273:1360); not at night, not in traf-
fic, but w someone else, on familiar roads; take driver's test w
copilot (J Am Ger Soc 1996;44:815); emphasize family's need to
develop clear plan for driving cessation—a necessary eventual
goal

- Ethical considerations: if demented pts unable to carry out decisions and manage their consequences, the presumption in favor
of maintaining autonomy as long as possible may need to be
reconsidered (J Am Ger Soc 1995;43:1437); 80% of elderly want
to be told about their dx of Alzheimer's disease vs 92% want to
be told of a terminal illness of medical origin (J Am Ger Soc
1996;44:404)

Discussion w pt and family including advanced directives (living
will, Durable Power of Attorney for Health Care) early on;
refer to local Alzheimer's chapter (J Gerontol Nurs 1983;9:
93); at end stage of disease: discuss "do not resuscitate"
(DNR), hospice; reassure that DNR does not mean "do not
treat" (Clin Ger Med 1994;10:91); be certain to establish
who has DPOA-HC and family "communication tree" in crisis; aim for acute illness care plan that is NH-centered as
much as possible, emphasizing risk issues w hospitalization
(worsening of cognition, disorientation, lack of understanding
by hospital staff)

NORMAL-PRESSURE HYDROCEPHALUS

Nejm 1985;312:1255

Cause: Idiopathic, postsurgical, trauma, subarachnoid hemorrhage, infectious meningitis, small-vessel disease

Pathophys: A "communicating hydrocephalus" (in contrast to foraminal or aqueductal), and obstruction is therefore at cisterna; hence, 4th ventricle may dilate causing cerebellar si's

Sx: First, trouble walking (ataxia problems with initiation and spasticity in lower extremity, leading to "magnetic gait," feet grip floor, only lifted with difficulty), progressive dementia, and incontinence; dementia includes psychomotor slowing, impaired ability to concentrate, mild memory difficulties

Si: Horizontal nystagmus, normal disks, spasticity, frontal lobe si's

Crs: Progressive dementia

Lab: CSF: transient but consistent improvement with removal of 50 mL (Acta Neurol Scand 1987;75:566) 1–3× in 1 wk; some neurosurgeons now not doing shunt unless see improvement with this first; Miller Fisher test—objective gait assessments before and after removal 30 mL CSF (Acta Neurol Scand 1986;73:566)

Xray: CT scan shows big ventricles (100%); cisternogram shows delayed or no movement of dye out over hemispheres, but there are false-neg results

Rx: Surgical shunt, 80% success (Nejm 1985;312:1255)

Cmplc: Infections in 3%–5%; factors associated with pos outcomes from shunting: short duration, known cause (trauma, hemorrhage), gait disturbance before onset of dementia or incontinence, presence of high-amplitude waves on intracranial pressure monitoring (Jama 1996;44:445)

VASCULAR DEMENTIAS

Cause:
1. Multiple subcortical (lacunar) or cortical infarctions (MID)
2. Ischemic demyelinization subcortical white matter—Binswanger's disease—clinical picture similar to MID
3. Single infarction; stroke not always leads to dementia (J Neurol Sci 1968;7:331); generally takes large amount brain tissue destroyed (J Neurol Sci 1970;11:205)

Epidem: Estimates of prevalence vary:

15% of all postmortem diagnosed dementias are vascular dementias; more common in blacks, Japanese (Neurol 1995;45:1161); MID overdiagnosed, needs more neuropathic correlation (Neurol 1993; 43:243); stroke frequently coexists w Alzheimer's or Parkinson's dementia (Arch Neurol 1989,46:651); estimated number of vascular dementias inflated when Hachinski index (point system based on presence of neurologic and atherosclerotic disease) used (47%–60%) (Nejm 1993;328:153)

Low prevalence MID 25% (Jama 1989;262:2551; Psychol Med 1990;20:881; J Neurol Sci 1990;95:239; Ann Neurol 1988;24:50; Alzheimer Dis Assoc Disord 1992;6:35)

Half of community-dwelling demented elderly have vascular dementia (Nejm 1993;328:153)

Pathophys: Amyloid deposits in walls of small cerebral blood vessels

Sx: Subcortical infarctions (basal ganglia, internal capsule, thalamus): slowness, forgetfulness, apathy, executive skill deficit; depression, anxiety; behavioral retardation more severe in pts w vascular dementia than in Alzheimer's

Si: Need temporal relationship between stroke and dementia to make dx vascular dementia (Neurol 1992;42:473; 1993;43:250; Nejm 1993;328:153); mixed 10%–20% of time

Erkinjuntti criteria for vascular dementia (NINDS-AIREN, Fortschr Neurol Psychiatrie 1994;62:197):

1. Focal neurologic signs + imaging findings: multiple lacunae (multiple motor and sensory deficits, rigidity, extrapyramidal signs, pseudobulbar palsy), extensive white matter lesions, multiple large-vessel infarcts strategically placed (angular gyrus, thalamus, basal forebrain)

2. Neurologic deficit and confusion occur within 3 mo of each other

3. Stepwise progression: ? dx utility of a hx of "stepwise progression," eg, episodic behavioral complications of Alzheimer's, eg, UTI may cause deterioration in behavior (Am J Psychiatry 1990;147:435)

Crs: Mortality from vascular dementia is higher; as more older people have strokes and survive, we will see more vascular dementia

Xray: CT: lacunar infarcts 50% of time w MID; MRI: Binswanger's: confluent deep white matter hyperintensities, periventricular white matter lesions (in nl aging too); central atrophy, 3rd ventricle enlargement marker for vascular dementia (Neurol 1995;45:1456)

Rx:

Preventive: Prevent and postpone atheromatosis and embolization through dietary changes and smoking cessation, aspirin, ? pentoxifylline; ticlopidine, HT control (may actually reverse cognitive impairment by treating preexisting HT) (J Am Ger Soc 1996;44: 411), DM, Afib management (Nejm 1993;328:153), anticoagulants; metabolic enhancing agents have not produced consistent benefits

SCHIZOPHRENIA (PARAPHRENIA)

Nurs Home Med 1995;3:248; J Am Ger Soc 1980;8:193; Schizophr Bull 1993;19:701,817

Cause: Sensory impairment debatable

Epidem: 0.1% in pts >65 yr old; 2%–12% of NH pts carry the diagnosis of new-onset schizophrenia; two-thirds of early-onset schizophrenic pts are left w mild symptoms by old age; M/F = 1:10 in elderly, ? estrogen protective

Pathophys: Dorsal lateral prefrontal cortex, superior temporal gyrus, hippocampus, basal ganglia

Sx: Pos or neg lasting for more than 6 mo; pos: delusions, hallucinations, distorted language and communication patterns, disorganized or catatonic behavior; neg: restriction in range, intensity of emotional expression, changes in fluency and productivity of thought and speech, changes in initiative; five categories: paranoid, disorganized, catatonic, undifferentiated, residual type; associated with schizoid premorbid personality, few surviving children, deafness, low socioeconomic class, female

Si: Difficulty focusing attention, formulating concepts, slowing in reaction time; cognitive impairments in memory and construction typical of Alzheimer's dementia not usual w paraphrenia

Crs: Paranoid delusions w or w/o hallucinations, usually with preservation of personality and affective response

Cmplc: R/o dementia, intracranial masses, thyroid disease, infections, liver disease, substance abuse, NPH, delirium, mania, depression

Lab:

Xray: CT, MRI: ventricular enlargement, cortical prominence, decreased temporal and hippocampal size, increased basal ganglia size; 5%–10% have lesions due to stroke

Rx:

> **Therapeutic:** Responsiveness to neuroleptics may be more favorable than in younger schizophrenics, risperidone 0.5 mg bid up to 4 mg/d and may respond to as little as 0.25 mg bid
>
> **Team Management:**
>
> *Nursing Home:* Make sure to obtain psychiatric records (should be a requirement for admission); identify neuroleptics taken within 2–4 wk; refer to Alzheimer's management

6. Infection

LUNG

PNEUMONIA

Cause: Community acquired: often more than one pathogen; streptococcal pneumonia still No. 1; TB in pts >60 yr old often with co-pathogens: *Streptococcus pneumoniae, Staphylococcus aureus, Haemophilus influenzae*, aerobic gram-neg bacilli, aerobes and anaerobes (aspiration), *Moraxella catarrhalis, Legionella pneumophila*

NH-acquired organisms of aspiration: *S. pneumoniae, Klebsiella pneumoniae, S. aureus, H. influenzae, Escherichia coli, M. catarrhalis, Mycobacterium tuberculosis; chlamydia pneumoniae* cause of rapid spread of respiratory infection in (Jama 1997;277:1214)

Hospital-acquired infection: aerobic gram-neg including *Pseudomonas aeruginosa*, like organisms of aspiration, *S. pneumoniae. S. aureus, H. influenzae, Legionella* (Am Rev Respir Dis 1993;148:14118); *S. aureus* and *S. pneumoniae* most common sequelae to influenza

Epidem: Pneumonia is the leading cause of death from infectious disease in the elderly (Geriatrics 1991;46:25); 11% pneumonia cases, but 85% pneumonia deaths in pts >65 yr old (Mmwr 1991;40:7); age alone doubles risk of complications and death; risk increases over 100× with each additional comorbid factor, especially CHF, COPD (Am J Med 1990;88(5N):1N; ANN IM 1991;115:428)

Pathophys: Age-related changes: decreased immunity, decreased cough and gag reflexes, decreased ciliary activity, increased colonization with resistant gram-neg organisms; comorbid diseases affecting ability to swallow such as strokes increase risk of aspiration pneumonia; 25% of all clinically septic pts (not just from pneumonia) are afebrile due to modified IL-1 response, hypothalamic alterations

Sx: Typical: shaking chill, fever, cough; decreased function (including cognition), falls, anorexia, 10% no symptoms; <35% typical presentation (J Am Ger Soc 1989;37:867); 50% of febrile geriatric pts presenting to ER w no other physical signs have serious illness including pneumonia

Si: Typical: rhonchi, rales, tachypnea; confusion (33% in community-acquired pneumonia vs 53% in NH–J Am Ger Soc 1986;34:697), tachypnea and dehydration, decreased function, anorexia, worsening of preexisting disease like CHF or COPD

Crs: Dx may be delayed with "atypical presentation"; this and comorbidities may contribute to longer course of illness, longer hospitalization in the elderly

Cmplc: Delayed resolution, bacteremia (40% mortality), death, mixed infections; r/o other infections, COPD, pulmonary embolus (PE), malignancy, drug reactions, myelodysplastic syndrome

Lab:
- *CBC*—important to compare w wbc baseline (20%–40% of all septic pts including from pneumonia do not develop leukocytosis–Ger Rev Syllabus 1996 p. 264)
- Electrolytes
- Oxygen saturation (use early and often in NH) to assess severity; if requiring hospital admission, then consider ABGs, blood culture, sputum Gram stain and culture (often impossible to obtain adequate sample, <50% can produce dx specimen) (Am J Med 1990; 88(5N):1N; J Am Ger Soc 1989;37:867)
- Urinary antigen for legionella; thoracentesis with stain and culture if significant pleural fluid present (Postgrad Med 1996;99(1))
- EKG

Xray: Chest film with infiltrate, though may not be obvious in setting of chronic lung changes

Rx: About two-thirds will require hospitalization; may be able to avoid hospital with risks of delirium, depression, and nosocomial infection if there is adequate NH or home care and the pt is hemodynamically stable; in some cases, the elderly and their families elect to have no further hospital care; consult advance directives for rx guidance; antibiotics, initially empiric broad-spectrum and then treat appropriate organism if becomes known; oxygen if indicated by decreased oxygen saturation or by clinical respiratory distress

Prevention: Influenza vaccine annually; pneumonia vaccine every 6 yr

Therapeutic: Oral outpatient or NH regimens include erythromycin, azithromycin, clarithromycin, amoxicillin–clavulanic acid, Tm/S, or a 2nd- or 3rd-generation cephalosporin or Tm/S (up to 24% *S. pneumoniae* resistance)

If hypoxic, serious underlying illness, or lives alone, cover *S. aureus* and gram-neg bacilli w iv ceftriaxone or im in NH pts w no iv access, along with oral or iv erythromycin or azithromycin for initial broad coverage; clindamycin is used when suspicion of anaerobic organisms is high

Hospital-acquired infection: iv β-lactam–β-lactamase inhibitor combination, or 3rd-generation cephalosporin and clindamycin or piperacillin

S. pneumoniae sens: 100%—vancomycin; 99.2%—ceftriaxone, doxycycline, levofloxacin; 99%—imipenem; 98.8%—erythromycin; 97.2%—ofloxacin; 96.2%—ciprofloxacin; 95%—cefuroxime; by 1994 increasing resistance developed including against penicillin (14%), ceftazadine (12%), and Tm/S (24%) (Jama 1996;275:194; Nejm 1996;335:1445)

Team Management: Caregiver awareness of baseline to recognize changes; community and institutional efforts to provide appropriate vaccinations and chemoprophylaxis for influenza and pneumonia; use acute crisis to focus future advance directive discussions, particularly w NH pts

INFLUENZA

Cause: Influenza virus, types A, B, C

Epidem: Worldwide: 90% of deaths associated with influenza are among those >65 yr old

Pathophys: RNA single-stranded viruses spread by respiratory droplets

Sx: Typical: cough, fever, malaise, sore throat, aches

Si: Typical: cough; geriatric: exacerbation of cardiopulmonary or chronic illness, changes in behavior/cognition

Crs: Incubation time only 1–2 d, symptoms usually last 5–6 d, malaise up to 2 wk

Cmpls: Primary influenza pneumonia, secondary bacterial pneumonia, and exacerbation of cardiopulmonary and other chronic illnesses result in increased hospitalization and death

R/o other viral URIs (Mmwr 1996;45:1)

Lab: Serology on first few cases to establish the type and strain of an outbreak

Xray: Chest film if secondary pneumonia suspected (threshold should be low to xray)

Rx:

    Prevention: Influenza vaccine annually for those >65 and/or working, living in institutional settings, or in elderly community (Ann IM 1995;123:518); each trivalent influenza vaccine usually includes two inactivated A strains and one B strain chosen each year based on observation of the antigenic characteristics of circulating strains during the previous season; new vaccine combination is required each year because of ongoing change (antigenic drift), so that immunity to last year's strains is unlikely to provide adequate protection from new variants in subsequent years

Pneumococcal vaccine should be given every 6 yr to those >65 yr old and should decrease incidence of secondary bacterial pneumonia; may give pneumococcal vaccine at the same time as influenza vaccine without problems; repeat every 6 yr as immunity already shown to wane after 5 yr

In the frail elderly, the vaccine may only prevent influenza infection 30%–40% of the time, but the severity of the illness is blunted; in NHs, influenza vaccination prevents an estimated 50%–60% of hospitalizations and pneumonia and 80% of deaths; influenza vaccine can decrease the hepatic metabolism of drugs including theophylline and warfarin, by 50% for up to a week; for those with contraindications of influenza vaccine, such as allergy to eggs or other vaccine components, the antiviral agents amantadine and rimantadine may be used prophylactically during the peak of the influenza season in a community

Amantadine or rimantadine should be started at the first indication of an influenza A outbreak in an institutional setting, even if pts have had the flu shot, for at least a 2-wk course or until 1 wk after the outbreak is over; initiation of amantadine or rimantidine within 48 h of the start of outbreak decreases the infection rate of influenza A by 70%–80%

    Therapeutic: Approach to fever in NH: fever >100°F for all infections including influenza (J Am Ger Soc 1996;44:74); antiviral resistant strains have emerged and can be shed as soon as the end of one rx course, dosages for those >65 are the same for prophylaxis and rx:

- Amantadine 100 mg po qd for those with creatinine clearance >50; adjust as per package insert for creatinine clearance <50
- Rimantadine 200 mg po qd, 100 mg po qd for creatinine clearance <10 or liver disease; observe carefully and decrease dose if CNS side effects noted; may increase seizure activity

Team Management: Caregiver awareness of baseline to recognize changes in clinical status; efficient administration of influenza vaccine and chemoprophylaxis in NH, boarding home, and community settings; caregiver, staff awareness of personal need for flu shot

PULMONARY TUBERCULOSIS

MacLennan WJ, Infection in the elderly, Little, Brown, 1995

Cause: Reactivation, crossinfection in NHs

Epidem: 8% conversion rate in 2½ yr in NH (Nejm 1985;312:1483); more at risk for reactivation w DM, alcoholism, smoking, cancer, partial gastrectomy, corticosteroids

Pathophys: Inhaled droplets containing microorganisms from untreated persons deposited in alveoli most commonly in lower lobes, replicate slowly, spread to regional lymph nodes in chest, then hematogenous spread; may have bronchopneumonia w initial infection but more often pts develop asx nodule (Ghon complex); TB reactivation occurs at sites w high oxygen concentration (upper lobes) because TB is an obligate aerobe, but mid and lower lobes can be involved in NH pts

Sx: May not have fever or night sweats; weight loss, cough, shortness of breath more common

Si: Pleural effusion

Crs: ARDS if miliary spread occurs, segmental atelectasis upper lobe; involvement of lingula or middle lobe can be mistaken for tumor

Complc: 10% of primary infections may progress to chronic TB or death (ascribed to antibiotic-unresponsive pneumonia); dissemination bone marrow, liver, gu tract, bone (spine = Pott's disease)

Lab: Polymorphonuclear leukocytosis, normocytic anemia, elevated ESR; examine 3 sputum samples for AFB, may take up to 12 wk to grow on culture medium (may be inhibited by ciprofloxacin, gentamicin, and amoxicillin-clavulanate (Augmentin)); pleural effusions may not reveal organisms

Xray: Delayed resolution of supposed bacterial infiltrate; classic findings of apical cavitary lesions less common; opacities of middle and upper lobes in isolation or w apical lesions more common; cavitation less common because of decreased cellular immunity

Rx:

Preventive: See screening (p 47)

Therapeutic: Treat NH residents w INH (300 mg/d) and rifampin (600 mg/d) for 9 mo because no multidrug resistance; 4-drug therapy reduces rx duration from 9 to 6 mo; first 2 mo:

- INH (300 mg): 5% develop hepatitis; 100 mg pyridoxine to avoid peripheral neuropathy; multiple drug interactions
- Rifampin (450 mg if pt <50 kg or 600 if pt >50 kg): 3% hepatitis; 8% hepatitis when taken in combination w INH; skin rash, gi sx; thrombocytopenia (uncommon); induces hepatic microenzymes
- Ethambutol (15 mg/kg): modify dosage in renal impairment to avoid retrobulbar neuritis (reduced visual acuity, scotomata, red, green color blindness); good synergistic action w rifampin against resistant mycobacteria
- Pyrazinamide (1.5 gm if <50 kg or 2 gm if >50 kg): 2%–6% hepatitis (dose-related), arthralgia, anorexia, nausea, photosensitivity, gout
- Streptomycin: high toxicity (vestibular, renal)
- Treat in hospital until smear-neg

HEART

ENDOCARDITIS

MacLennan WJ, Infection in the elderly, Little, Brown, 1995

Cause: Etiology of septicemia found in <50% of pts, prosthetic valves; pacemakers; *S. aureus* can cause endocarditis in a preexisting healthy valve

Epidem: More than one-half of pts w endocarditis are elderly because they have more prosthetic valves, hospital-acquired bacteremia, rheumatic valvular lesions

Pathophys: Alteration in endothelial surface, deposition platelets and fibrin, vegetation where there is increased turbulence; Streptococcus 25%–70%, *Streptococcus bovis* 25% (associated w gi malignancy, especially colon cancer), staphylococcus 20%–30%, enterococcus from gu 25%, *Streptococcus viridans* less common than in younger pts; culture neg 10%–20%

Sx: Aortic and mitral valve regurgitation most common, heart failure, systemic embolism, cerebral embolism (25% of time presenting as acute confusional state)

Si: Suspect in pts w pyrexia, high ESR, CHF, peripheral emboli, vaguely unwell after recent gi or gu procedure, changing cardiac murmur; still suspect w pos blood cultures despite no heart murmur; may see splenomegaly w *S. viridans;* Janeway's lesions on palms and soles and Roth's spots on fundi indicative of emboli; immune complexes produce Osler's nodes, arthralgias, finger clubbing, petechiae, glomerulonephritis, hematuria

Crs: 50% mortality

Cmplc: R/o myocardial abscess if ESR does not come down w rx or LBBB, or progressive lengthening of PR interval

Lab: 3 blood cultures establish cause in 95% of pts, *S. viridans* (30%–45%), assoc w dental procedure, not all penicillin-sens; staphylococcus (10%–30%) coagulase-neg associated w prosthetic valves, better prognosis than with *S. aureus;* other streptococci (10%–15%) include enterococci (*S. bovis*)

Associated w colon cancer and diverticulosis, gu manipulation in men, varying resistance

ESR >100 mm/h, elevated C-reactive protein acute-phase reactant, 50% rheumatoid factor, and ANA positive, normochromic normocytic anemia, elevated wbc

Xray:

Noninvasive: Echocardiography (transthoracic and transesophageal): vegetations on prosthetic valves, septal or annular abscess; two-dimensional echocardiography allows evaluation of chamber size and serial evaluations can be done if worsening valve dysfunction; if neg and still suspect clinically, recheck echocardiogram

Rx:

Preventive (Nejm 1995;332:38): For pts w cardiac disorders (highest risk w prosthetic valves, previous infective endocarditis, aortic regurgitation, aortic stenosis, mitral stenosis and regurgitation, s/p intracardiac surgery w residual hemodynamic abnormality)

For procedures involving mouth or respiratory tract: amoxicillin 23 gm po 1 h before procedure (Jama 1997;277:1794)

Manipulation of gu or gi tract (enterococcus): 1 gm ampicillin and 1.5 mg/kg, not to exceed (Jama 1997;277:1794) 120 mg gentamicin iv 1 h before procedure and 6 h later; ampicillin lg IM/IV or amoxicillin lg po; if penicillin-allergic, substitute 1 gm vancomycin

Prevent hospital-acquired infection

Prosthetic valves (staphylococcus): use regimen for enterococcus

Therapeutic (Table 6-1): Doses that reach bactericidal concentrations; EKG to follow clinical course; surgery may be needed if worsening CHF, embolism, cardiac abscess, vegetations >10 mm

Table 6-1. Treatment for Endocarditis

Organism	Treatment
Streptococci	MIC <0.1 mg/L (= high sens), give benzylpenicillin 20 million units over 24 h, may have to use ampicillin if high sodium load compromises cardiac function; if MIC >0.1 mg/L, add aminoglycoside for synergistic effect × 2–4 wk (trough levels = 2–3 mg/L to achieve synergy, reduce risk of renal and ototoxicity); if cardiac abscess, continue penicillin 2 wk past the cessation of aminoglycoside; if prosthetic valve, continue the penicillin for 4 wk, then switch to amoxicillin po fo 2 wk; penallergic, use vancomycin 15 mg/kg 12 hourly, but is ototoxic and renal toxic
Enterococci	Penicillin-resistant, but if give penicillin and gentamicin, they are synergistic and can be given together in an iv infusion
Staphylococci	Oxacillin or nafcillin 2 gm iv q 4 h × 6 wk; coagulase-neg staphylococci involve prosthetic valves and are often β-lactam resistant, give vancomycin and gentamicin; MRSA treated in same way; replace prosthesis once infection has been stabilized w 2-wk course of antibiotics; if infection associated w pacemaker, remove catheter and treat w antibiotics for 6 wk w outpatient parenteral therapy (Hosp Prac 1993;28(suppl 2, part II)

MIC = minimal inhibitory concentration; MRSA = methicillin-resistant *S. aureus.*

or fungal infection; valve replacement delayed until residual infection of valve annulus, adjacent structures reduced; anticoagulation not much help

BONES AND JOINTS

OSTEOMYELITIS/SEPTIC ARTHRITIS/JOINT PROSTHESIS INFECTION

MacLennan WJ, Infection in the elderly, Little, Brown, 1995; Nejm 1997;336:999

Cause:
- Septic arthritis: chronic septic arthritis most often caused by staphylococcus
- Joint prosthesis infection: staphylococcus, gram-neg, anaerobes

Epidem:
- Septic arthritis: 25%–33% in pts >60 yr old; impaired immune system; preexisting joint disease, eg, osteoarthritis and rheumatoid arthritis; staphylococcus, streptococcus, gram-neg bacteria; hematogenous spread from UTI, cellulitis, endocarditis, salmonella bowel infections; predisposing factors: malnutrition, diabetes, chronic renal failure, hepatic cirrhosis, malignancy, alcoholism, corticosteroids
- Joint prosthesis infection: 1%–2%, hematogenous spread from surgery; sources: gums, gi tract, urinary tract

Sx:
- Septic arthritis: tenderness, redness, warmth, diabetics may not have pain or pyrexia, may just see blood glucose values out of control and gradual onset; normocytic normochromic anemia
- Chronic septic arthritis: may not have pyrexia or tachycardia, just sinus tract

Si:
- Osteomyelitis: foot: metatarsal heads, proximal phalanges, close to ulcer discharging pus from a sinus; erythema and swelling over infected bone; fluctuant swelling, painful limitation of active and passive movement, usually febrile; difficult to diagnose w preex-

isting joint disease; masked in sternoclavicular, sacroiliac, hips, and shoulder joints

Cmplc:

- Septic arthritis: osteomyelitis in adjacent bones, avascular necrosis, septicemia, high mortality; chronic septic arthritis: bacteremia common, giving rise to endocarditis, cholecystitis, cerebral abscess (high mortality approaching 50%)

Lab:

- Osteomyelitis: blood cultures pos in 50% pts w hematogenous osteomyelitis; culture discharging sinuses w sterile syringe; bone bx; elevated wbc, high ESR may not be present in the elderly
- Septic arthritis: only 50% elderly have elevated wbc; ESR usually elevated; large-bore needle w heparin to prevent clotting for joint tap: wbc = 100,000/μL in half the pts, 90% polymorphonuclear leukocytes, elevated lactate, culture pos in <two-thirds pts
- Joint prosthesis infection: blood cultures

Xray:

- Osteomyelitis: initial phases on xray show soft tissue swelling over the diaphysis indistinguishable from changes w cellulitis; 2 wk after onset: translucency of the cortex of the diaphysis, radiopaque new bone formation under an elevated periosteum, sclerosis anytime after 3 wk

In elderly pts periosteum more likely to be adherent to cortex, so infection does not separate the bone layers; gallium scan to define areas of chronic or subacute infection; CT and MRI to distinguish osteomyelitis from soft tissue infection; MRI less useful in infections related to surgical pins

If the vertebral arch is involved, underlying process is malignant; osteoporosis may mask areas of lysis; MRI pos in vertebral osteomyelitis 95% of the time

- Septic arthritis: radionucleotide scan for less accessible joints: hips, sacroiliacs
- Joint prosthesis infection: translucency of surrounding bone; technetium and gallium scans helpful in late infection; US in detection of abscess?

Rx:

Therapeutic:

- Osteomyelitis: 3 wk antibiotics minimum to prevent progression to chronic osteomyelitis, oral therapy should be started 24 h before cessation of iv antibiotics

Chronic osteomyelitis: treat for several months; methicillin-resistant *S. aureus* may respond to clindamycin, erythromycin, rifampin, but vancomycin may be required; gram-neg, eg, pseudomonas: quinolones (especially chronic); anaerobic osteomyelitis: metronidazole; osteomyelitis difficult to treat w trauma or vascular insufficiency: often requires surgical intervention

- Septic arthritis: iv antibiotics for at least 6 wk, intra-articular injections of no benefit; benzylpenicillin, and aminoglycosides do not achieve adequate levels in joints; surgical debridement and exploration may be needed, especially w hip involvement
- Joint prosthesis infection: early: 3 wk antibiotics may avoid losing the prosthesis; late: remove prosthesis, pack w antibiotic-impregnated cement and begin parenteral antibiotics × 6 wk; persistent in 60% pts

  Preventive:
- Joint prosthesis infection: 24 h before surgery use prophylactic antibiotics (J Bone Joint Surg Am 1990;72:1); treat mouth, alimentary, and gu infections prior to surgery

---

CENTRAL NERVOUS SYSTEM

MENINGITIS

See Table 6-2

SKIN

Young EM, Geriatric dermatology, Lea & Febiger, 1993

Cause: Thinning epidermis, decreased sebaceous gland secretion compromises barrier between sc tissue and external environment; less effective T-cell immunity

Pathophys, sx, si, crs, lab, rx:
See Table 6-3

Table 6-2. Meningitis

Organism	Si/sx	Crse/complc	Lab	Rx
Bacterial				
Pneumococcus	Rapid coma, convulsions	Subdural empyema, cerebral vein or sinus thrombosis, middle cerebral arteritis causing hemiparesis; permanent memory deficit, NPH	Increased PMNLs, glucose >45 mg/dL, protein <45 mg/dL	Penicillin (up to 24 gm/d), or vancomycin plus broad-spectrum cephalosporin (resistant organisms)
Meningococcus	Septicemia, acute confusional state, agitation, aggression	Deafness often permanent, transient paralysis of 6th and 7th CNs	Increased PMNLs, glucose >45 mg/dL, protein <45 mg/dL	Penicillin G or cefuroxime
Staphylococci	Sequela to infection elsewhere or shunt procedure	50%–75% mortality	Increased PMNLs, glucose >45 mg/dL, protein <45 mg/dL	Oxacillin, w rifampin; or vancomycin
Gram-negative	After head injury, in pts w DM, cancer, cirrhosis	—	Increased PMNLs, glucose >45 mg/dL, protein <45 mg/dL	3rd-generation cephalosporin, plus aminoglycoside (Nejm 1997;336:703) *H. influenzae:* ceftriaxone
Viral meningoercephalitis herpes simplex type 1	Primary or reactivation infection headache, fever, neck stiffness; personality change; dysphagia; impaired temperature regulation, abnormal bladder function, postural hypotension	(Stroke syndrome—ipsilateral middle cerebral artery to ophthalmic involvement)	CSF: lymphocytosis up to 1000/μL, rbc's, glucose nl, protein mildly elevated; acute, convalescent titers; temporal lobe abnormalities on EEG, CT, MRI after 6 d obtundation, neurologic deficit	—

Table 6-3. Skin Infections

Disease	Path / Sx / Si / Crs / Lab	Rx
Bacterial		
Cellulitis	Red, tender, warm, swollen, fever, elevated wbc, ESR; distinguish it from DVT	Amoxicillin or amoxicillin–clavulanate potassium to cover group A streptococci, *S. aureus;* metronidazole for anaerobes
Erysipelas	Variant of cellulitis w well-demarcated borders, patches of hemorrhage, exudate, and bullous erruption on leg; β-hemolytic strep, *S. aureus;* recur in 2–4 yr; higher risk w peripheral edema	Benzylpenicillin 600 mg im bid 2–3 d then po penicillin; dicloxacillin or amoxicillin–clavulanate potassium for *S. aureus*
Furunculosis	Tender red nodule that develops into pustule, abscess in hair follicle, may recur in areas of excessive sweating, restrictive clothing; diabetes risk factor	Drain, antibiotics for *S. aureus,* occasional anaerobes, shampoo and bath w chlorhexidine; if nasal carrier of staph, use bacitracin or mupirocin
Impetigo	Cutaneous inflammation w honey-colored crusts	Treat *S. aureus* w dicloxacillin 250 mg qid or topically w mupirocin 2%
Fungal		
Candidiasis	Glazed red skin w satellite lesions; intertrigenous; beneath condom catheters, around stomas, fistulas; spread to the fingers by scratching; chronic paronychia w loss of cuticle and brawny swelling	2% miconazole bid × 2–3 wk; nystatin ointment or imidazole cream in nail fold several times a day
Onchomycosis	Thickening, irregularity, and discoloration of toe nail	Treat selectively; podiatry consult for mechanical improvements and to reduce nail mass; terbinafine po 125 mg bid, resolution in 6 mo, mild gl side effects (Lancet 1990; 1:636), griseofulvin, ketoconazole (Nizoral)

Table 6-3. *(Continued)*

Disease	Path / Sx / Si / Crs / Lab	Rx
Fungal 　Tinea	Dermatophytosis—annular red brown patches on scalp, face, extremities; candidiasis—beefy red patches thick white coating; T. versicolor—white tan confluent macules on upper trunk; dermatophytid reaction—allergic vesicles on palm or finger after exposure to fungus	T. pedis, cruris, corporus: astringent aluminum acetate solution (Domeboro), 1% tolnaftate, clotrimazole, griseofulvin; capitus, versicola: 2.5% selenium sulfide; barbis: fluconazole 2% × 2–3 d
Scabies	Sarcoptes mite burrows into skin, laying eggs causing immune response and intense itching; seldom on face, commonly axilla, waist, inner thighs, back, arms, legs, web spaces fingers; few mm long linear raised burrow	Eurax—wash off 24 h after application; itch may continue 2 wk after rx; launder and heat dry clothing and bedding
Burns	—	1% Sulfadiazine-silver (Silvadene)—dicloxacillin 250 mg po q 6 h for staph, strep; quinolone for *P. aeruginosa*
Pressure ulcers	—	Prophylactic antibiotics produce resistant organisms; antiseptics, eg, povidine-iodine, may be helpful; 0.5% acetic acid for wounds infected w *P. aeruginosa*
Herpes virus 　Simplex types 1, 2	Small patch of blisters involving skin and mucosa, lip, gums, and hard palate, can present as exema, can involve eye; herpetic Whitlow, fingers; rarely elsewhere on body	Acyclovir topically; acyclovir oral (400 mg tid × 7–10 d) may help—intermittent use

Table 6-3. *(Continued)*

Disease	Path / Sx / Si / Crs / Lab	Rx
Zoster	Malaise, paresthesias affecting single root dermatome precede papular rash which becomes vesicular, sometimes hemorrhagic; reactiation of chicken pox virus: duration 2–3 wk–many mo; trigeminal nerve distribution, cornea, iris; lesion on tip nose = risk for ophthalmic involvement; overlapped dermatomes = disseminated; postherpetic neuralgia 50%	Rx within 48 h of rash w acyclovir 800 mg 5 × a day for 7 d speeds recovery but effective only early in course, does not prevent postherpetic neuralgia; corticosteroids not help postinfective neuralgia; can try amitriptyline (Elavil) 10 mg, carbamazepine (Tegretol), capsaicin topical ointment, or TENS; not contagious once crusted over; extent of contagiousness debated, but caution and covering of active skin lesions advised

GASTROINTESTINAL TRACT

See Table 6-4

EYE

CONJUNCTIVITIS

See Table 6-5

HUMAN IMMUNODEFICIENCY VIRUS INFECTION

Nurs Home Med 1995;3:265; J Am Ger Soc 1995;43:7; Arch IM 1994; 154:57; 1995;155:184; Geriatrics 1993;48:61; J Comm Health 1995;20:383; J Acquir Immun Defic Syndr 1991;4:84
Cause: HIV
Epidem: 10% of pts w AIDS are >50 yr old (J Acquir Immun Defic

Table 6-4. Gastrointestinal Infections

Disease	Cause	Sx/si	Crse/complc	Lab	Rx
Oral Parotitis	Xerostomia, anticholinergics, malnutrition, DM	Swollen tender parotid gland, red warm overlying skin; pus expressed from Stenson's duct; patient may not complain of pain because symptoms may be masked by other infections (pneumonia, abdominal abscess)	Complc septicemia, osteomyelitis facial bones, facial nerve palsy; parotid abscess w rupture into pharynx or auditory canal, 10%–50% mortality	Commensal aerobic and anaerobic organisms in the floor of the mouth	iv cefuroxime w metronidazole or amoxiclavulinic acid until organism identified; discontinue anticholinergics; may need to drain w external excision
Candidiasis	Anemia, agranulocytosis; CRF; alcoholism; deficiency in riboflavin, nicotinic acid, ascorbic acid; DM, poor oral hygiene (dentures); antibiotics; steroids	Red, raw mucous membrane, w or w/o sheets of whitish pseudomembrane patches	—	Yeast budding cells and pseudohyphae on Gram stain	Nystatin pastilles 100 000 units qid or amphotericin lozenges 10 mg qid, or miconazole gel 10 mL qid p meals, retaining near lesion before swallowing; fluconazole 100 mg qd systemic therapy; chronic glossitis: coat dentures w nystatin ointment × 2 wk
Stomatitis	Medication side effect: furosemide, HCTZ, β-blockers, cholestyramine, desipramine, doxepine, ACE-inhibitors (J Am Ger Soc 1995;43:1414)	—	—	—	—

Table 6-4. *(Continued)*

Disease	Cause	Sx/si	Crse/complc	Lab	Rx
Dental abscess	Enterococcus (endocarditis), *S. pyogens* (glomerulonephritis), actinomycetes (cervicofacial, brain abscess)	—	—	—	—
Gingivitis	Peptostreptococcus (lung, brain abscess), gram negative rods (pneumonia, endocarditis) (J Am Ger Soc 1995;43:1414), calcium channel blockers	—	—	—	—
Peptic ulcer	*H. pylori*, atrophic gastritis, NSAIDs (see gastrointestinal diseases)	—	—	—	—
Small-bowel overgrowth	Achlorhydria, jejunal diverticular disease; surgery leading to blind loops, overgrowth of bacteria causes more metabolism of vit B_{12} resulting in B_{12} deficiency	Malabsorption, weight loss, diarrhea	Severe overgrowth can lead to protein-energy deficiency; bacteria synthesize folic acid so may see increase in folic acid levels; bacteroides cause deconjugation of bile salts and reduce solubility and absorption of lipids	Macrocytic anemia, ostomalacia, culture jejunal contents	Broad-spectrum antibiotics including metronidazole; surgical intervention

Diarrhea		R/o noninfectious causes (diverticulosis, inflammatory bowel disease, ischemic colitis, bowel cancer, laxative, theophylline derivatives, NSAIDs, sulfa derivatives, iron supplements, levodopa, cimetidine, ranitidine, allopurinol	
Clostridium difficile 25% of antibiotic-associated diarrhea (ampicillin, amoxicillin, cephalosporins most common)	Varying causes of loose watery or frequent stools		Rx: *C. difficile* w vancomycin 125 mg q 6 h for 10 d, $\frac{1}{3}$ recur, rx w metronidazole, single room precautions
Campylobacter from inadequately prepared poultry	When severe explosive watery w blood and mucus; pyrexia, dehydration, and shock		*Campylobacter* when severe, use erythromycin
Salmonella from egg products	Incubation 2-3 d; colicky abdominal pain; diarrhea can be blood-stained	*Salmonella, shigella:* may be severe (bacteremia, septicemia) in elderly because of heavy inoculum; lower gi not protected by stomach acidity (achlorhydria); *Salmonella choleraesuis* causes endocarditis	*Salmonella:* always rx w antibiotics: ciprofloxacin 500 mg bid × 7 d or 14 d if bacteremia; or 200 iv bid at first w nausea
Shigella, fecal oral route direct contact	Incubation 3-24 h; vomiting, colic-like pain; watery diarrhea w blood or mucus; sometimes severe dehydration		Rx of *dehydration:* oral (Dextrolyte, Glucolyte, Rehidrat) 2-3 Lt; may be difficult in elderly because of impaired thirst and decreased response to ADH; then give 0.9% sodium chloride 3 L/d; avoid D$_5$ if Na >160 mmol/L
S. aureus, heat-labile enterotoxin eg, cold meats not recooked	Incubation 2-4 d, tenesmus; colicky abdominal pain; watery, bloody or mucus containing stool; elderly may get bacteremia		
Norwalk, rotavirus	Incubation few hours; vomiting; diarrhea: self-limiting		
	Vomiting, mild diarrhea 2-7 d self-limited; except rotavirus in NH can cause fatal dehydration		

CRF = chronic renal failure; ADH = antidiuretic hormone.
Adapted from MacLennon W. Infections in elderly people. Little, Brown, 1994.

Table 6-5. Conjunctivitis

	Itching	Tearing	Exudate	Periauricular Adenopathy
Viral	Minimal	+	Minimal (follicle formation) keratoconjunctivitis: subepithelial opacities in epidemics, 3–4 wk	+
Bacterial	Minimal	Moderate	+	Uncommon
Chlamydial	Minimal	Moderate	+	+
Allergic	+	Moderate	Minimal	None

+ = little or few.

Syndr 1991;4:84); 3% >60 yr old, expected to reach 10% within decade; risk factors—homosexual sex 45%, transfusion 20%, heterosexual sex 11%, iv drug abuse 8%, other 16%; pts age >50 less likely to use condoms; greatest risk is to not consider the dx in elderly pts with risk factors

Pathophys: HIV infection leading to progressive decreased immune function and subsequent opportunistic infections (Table 6-6)

Sx: Early—viral syndrome; late—dementia, AIDS dementia–subcortical

Table 6-6. HIV/AIDS Associated Diseases

Disease	T-cell Count	Time after Initial Exposure
Acute retroviral syndrome, oral, esophageal candidiasis	Dips to 600 cells/μL; returns to 1000 cells/μL within 1 mo	first 3–4 mo
Pneumococcal pneumonia, vaginal candidasis, idiopathic thrombocytopenic purpura	350–500 cells/μL	2–5 yr
Kaposi's sarcoma, oral candidiasis, lymphoma, TB, dementia	200–350 cells/μL	5–8 yr
Pneumocystis infection, cryptococcosis, histoplasmosis, coccidiomycosis	150–250 cells/μL	8–9 yr
Mycobacterium avium, cytomegalovirus	<100 cells/μL	10 yr

From HIV/AIDS Surveill Rep 1994;6:1.

type, rapidly progressive as compared to Alzheimer's type; often associated with peripheral neuropathies, myelopathies

Si: Can be nonspecific

Crs: Faster progression in elderly, w disease-free period being much less than 11 yr (San Francisco cohort)

Cmplc: Specific to opportunistic infection; AIDS dementia complex: mild abnormal on psychometric tests, inability to perform demanding job tasks, can perform ADLs; progressing to need for cane, then walker, wheelchair, then paraplegia in end stages; inability to work, upper extremity weakness, progressing to double incontinence, mutism, and vegetative cognitive state in end stages

Lab: Initial w/u as with other age groups; AIDS dementia often associated with elevated protein levels and relative monocytosis in CSF

Xray: Disease-specific (eg, PCP—chest film, serum LDH, ABG)

Rx:

> **Prevention:** Encourage condom use; therapy (protease inhibitors) may need to be initiated at lower doses secondary to decreased renal clearance in the elderly
>
> **Team Management:** Multidisciplinary; parenting by grandparents as a result of the AIDS epidemic is increasing

7. Hematology/Oncology

HEMATOLOGY

ANEMIAS

Ger Rev Syllabus 1996, p. 314

Cause: Hypoproliferative is the most common in elderly: Fe deficiency (blood loss), chronic diseases and inflammation, marrow damage or dysfunction, erythropoietin deficiency (renal, thyroid, nutritional)

Ineffective erythropoiesis: megaloblastic (vit B_{12}, folate), microcytic (thalassemia, sideroblastic), normocytic

Hemolytic anemia: immunologic (tumor, drug, collagen vascular, idiopathic), intrinsic (metabolic, abnormal hgb), extrinsic (mechanical, lytic substance)

Epidem: >33% outpatients, after age 85 more common in men (44%) (Mayo Clin Proc 1994;69:730)

Pathophys: Differential diagnosis: hypochromia (Figure 7-1)

Sequential changes in Fe deficiency begin w decrease in serum ferritin, followed by low serum Fe and increase in TIBC, then change in rbc indices and decreased hgb

Primary autonomic failure present in 38% of elderly w primary autonomic dysfunction (reduced erythropoietin secretion), decreased BP and compensatory increase in heart rate, 80% success w erythropoietin 50 units/kg 3×/wk (Ann IM 1994;121:181)

Myelodysplastic syndrome where hematopoietic precursors abundant but defective maturation and peripheral cells have shorter life span and can develop into CML; caused by alkylating agents, RNA virus, somatic mutations, radiation, environmental toxins; 20% in pts over 65 yr old and twice as common in men; anemia, thrombocytopenia, leukopenia presenting w fatigue, exercise intolerance, purpura, infection; hepatomegaly 5%, splenomegaly 10%, pallor 50%; find increased Fe stores, hemochromatosis, basophilic stip-

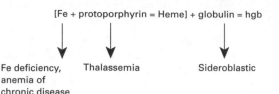

[Fe + protoporphyrin = Heme] + globulin = hgb

Fe deficiency, anemia of chronic disease   Thalassemia   Sideroblastic

Figure 7-1. Causes of anemia based on deficits in hemaglobin-molecule production.

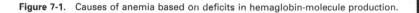

pling, monocytosis in 30%, elevated LDH; 3-yr mortality, better prognosis if only erythroid dysplasia

Sx: Fatigue, worsening shortness of breath, angina, peripheral edema related to underlying atherosclerotic heart disease; mental status changes, dizziness, poor balance, pallor less noticeable; commonly without sx if slow onset

Si: Fe deficiency causes atrophy of the tongue, buccal mucosa, angular stomatitis, atrophic gastritis which can lead to achlorhydria and vit B_{12} deficiency

Megaloblastic: glossitis, mild jaundice, paresthesias and abnormal position and vibratory senses, dementia, depression, mania

Crs: Megaloblastic stages: first vit B_{12} <300 pg/mL; then hypersegmented neutrophils; then anemia; neurologic damage and dementia seem to occur before hypersegmented phase

Lab:
- <11% hgb
- Check stool guaiac
- If reticulocyte count high, consider hemolysis (warm-reactive IgG or more commonly cold-reactive IgM); if reticulocyte count low, check rbc size:

  Check vit B_{12}, folate if macrocytic (anti-intrinsic factor antibodies, if can't obtain 24-h urine w Schilling test and if normal, obtain bone marrow aspirate)

  Check transferrin saturation if microcytic or normocytic:

  If transferrin nl (>20%), check hgb electrophoresis—fetal and $HgbA_2$ (thalassemia)

  If transferrin <20%, check TIBC, ferritin

  If TIBC <250 gm/dL, ferritin >100 ng/mL, anemia chronic disease, thyroid, renal

If TIBC >400 gm/dL, ferritin <20 ng/mL, Fe deficiency anemia
If TIBC 250–400 gm/dL, ferritin 20–100 ng/mL, check for
ringed sideroblasts, and Fe stores in marrow
Anemias may be "mixed" types in elderly (rbc distribution width
index elevated)

Rx:

Preventive: Dietary review routinely

Therapeutic: Chronic disease: erythropoietin 50–100 units/kg
3×/wk, increase dose to 150 units/kg if no response in 2–3 wk
(Nejm 1997;336:933)

Fe deficiency: ferrous sulfate 325 mg tid; start w 1 tab/d and build up
over 2 wk to avoid constipation; 6 mo needed to replenish Fe stores

Fe replacement contraindicated in thalassemia because produces Fe
overload

Hemolysis: remove offending drug, eg, levodopa, penicillin, doxepin,
quinidine, thiazides; rx IgG (warm) w prednisone 60 mg/d, dana-
zol, splenectomy, azothiaprine, cyclophosphamide, transfusion if
unstable, emergency—immunogobulin 0.4 gm/kg/d × 5 ds; rx
IgM (cold) w transfusion, plasmapheresis

Vit B_{12} 1000 µg/d orally until serum B_{12} >300 pg/mL or parenteral
1000 µg/d 1st wk × 4 then q mo; folic acid 1 mg/d

Myelodyplasia: rx w washed rbc's, granulocyte transfusion, antibiotics, blood cell products w hydroxyurea to keep wbc's down

Intermittent transfusion may be warranted occasionally, particularly
in anemia of chronic disease, if pt otherwise stable; will improve
quality of life

CHRONIC LYMPHOCYTIC LEUKEMIA

Ger Rev Syllabus 1996, p. 319; Nejm 1995;333:1032

Cause: No genes have been identified; 50% have cytogenetic abnormalities: trisomy 12, chromosome 13 at band q14

Epidem: Most common form of leukemia in Western countries

Pathophys: Accumulation of neoplastic B lymphocytes in blood, bone
marrow, liver, and spleen; monoclonal proliferation (Leukemia
1994;8:1610)

Sx: Fatigue; malaise; decreased exercise tolerance; exacerbation CAD, cardiovascular disease; abdominal pain; early satiety w splenomegaly; >25% asx

Si: Enlarged lymph nodes (cervical, axillary, supraclavicular); splenomegaly; hepatomegaly w disease progression; jaundice secondary to hemolysis or biliary obstruction from enlarged periportal lymph nodes; ecchymoses, petechiae in late stages secondary to thrombocytopenia; fever in late stages may be secondary to the development of lymphoma

Crs: 60% diagnosed in asx phase; staging worsens in the following order: lymphocytosis >50 000/μL, lymph node enlargement, splenomegaly, hgb <11 gm/dL, thrombocytopenia (platelet count <10^5/μL); life span varies from nl to 5 yr w median survival 9 yr

Cmplc: Hypogammaglobulinemia chief cause of infection (Leuk Lymphoma 1994;13:203)

Lab: Criteria: 95% small mature lymphocytes; bone marrow confirms

Xray:

Rx:

Therapeutic:

- Treat constitutional symptoms, bulky lymphadenopathy, splenomegaly causing compressive problems, doubling of wbc in under 1 yr: chlorambucil 0.4–0.8 mg/kg body weight po q 2 wk for 8–12 mo yielding response rates of 40%–70%; addition of prednisone no help; combination therapy does not prolong survival (Ann Oncol 1995;6:219); discontinue treatment when response has been achieved and restart w disease progression

- If no response due to gene mutation, try purine analogue, fludarabine (Blood 1994;84(suppl 1):461a.abstract)

- Treat pts w cytopenias w high-dose immunoglobulin, cyclosporine, splenectomy, low-dose radiation of the spleen

- Hypogammaglobulinemia not helped much by vaccines that produce a suboptimal response

- Neutropenia from chemotherapy can be treated w hematopoietic growth factors

- International Bone Marrow Transplant registry: probability 3-yr survival = 46% (Bone Marrow Transplant 1995;15(suppl 2):S11)

- Monoclonal antibodies for minimal residual disease (Ann Oncol 1995;6:219)

HEMATOLOGY, ONCOLOGY

MULTIPLE MYELOMA

J Am Ger Soc 1994;42:653

Cause: Proliferation of plasma cells and plasma cell precursors, usually monoclonal IgG or IgA; translocations 14 q 32 and chromosomes 11, 6, 16, 9, 18, 8; point mutations; monoclonal gamopathy representing 1st oncogenic event leads to multiple myeloma in 1690 cases over 30 yr period − a second oncogenic event (Nejm 1997; 336:1657)

Epidem: Mean age at diagnosis = 69.1 yr; black males highest incidence, 9.6 cases/100 000; increased risk w asbestos exposure, farming, atomic bomb survivors, radium dial workers

Pathophys: First loss of T cell–mediated control of early B-cell development, then abnormal proliferation of multiple clones, followed by malignant transformation, and accumulation of immunoglobulins typically produced by that clone; clinical manifestations result from tumor growth, accumulation of immunoglobulin chains, and cytokines released from malignant plasma cells (bone resorption)

Sx: 60%–70% of newly diagnosed pts have bone pain (Eur J Cancer 1991;27:1401); hypercalcemia: anorexia, nausea, vomiting, constipation, weakness, pain, confusion, and lethargy

Si:

Crs: Prognosis for healthy old people same as for healthy young people (Am J Med 1985;79:316) (Table 7-1)

Cmplc: Renal failure: up to one-half of pts have renal insufficiency at the time of diagnosis; light chains precipitate in renal tubules, leading to obstruction, dilatation, and subsequent atrophy of the nephron; other mechanisms renal dysfunction: amyloid, infection, hyperuricemia

Amyloid and hyperviscosity: results from deposition of immunoglobulin light chains in susceptible organs, eg, kidneys, gi tract, myocardium, peripheral nerves; manifestations of hyperviscosity: mucosal bleeding, retinopathy, CHF; sx may be absent in the setting of anemia, so use caution when deciding to transfuse

Hypogammaglobulinemia and infection: major cause of morbidity in multiple myeloma pts, increased risk w encapsulated organisms: *Streptococcus pneumoniae, Haemophilus influenzae, Staphylococcus aureus,* gram-neg rods (Semin Oncol 1986;13:282)

Table 7-1. Durie and Salmon Staging System

Stage	Criteria	Survival
I	All of following:	46 mo
	Hgb >10 gm/dL	
	Calcium <12 mg/dL	
	Normal bones or single plas-	
	macytoma	
	Low M component	
	a. IgG <5 gm/dL	
	b. IgA <3 gm/dL	
	c. Urinary M-component	
	<4 gm/24 h	
II	Neither stage I nor II	32 mo
III	Hgb <8.5 gm/dL	23 mo
	Calcium >12 mg/dL	
	Advanced bone disease	
	High M-component	
	a. IgG >7 gm/dL	
	b. IgA >5 gm/dL	
	c. Urinary M-component	
	>12 gm/24 h	
Subclassification		
A = serum Creatinine <2.0 mg/dl		32 mo
B = serum Creatinine >2.0 mg/dL		11 mo

From J Am Ger Soc 1994;42:653.

Lab: 10% atypical plasma cells in bone marrow, monoclonal immuno-globulin in serum, light chains in urine; Hgb <12 gm/dL; normo-cytic, normochromic w few reticulocytes; rouleaux formation because of excess monoclonal protein; identify in tissue w Congo red stain

Prognostic tests: β_2-microglobulin <4 µg/mL better prognosis; plasma cell labeling index is a measure of DNA replication and reflects tumor growth (Blood 1988;72:219); IL-6 levels are higher w severe disease (J Clin Invest 1989;84:2008); follow M protein on SPEP, UPEP; proteinuria; follow recurrence w β_2-microglobulin tumor marker

Xray: Multiple osteolytic lesions throughout skeleton, pathologic frac-tures, and osteopenia on xray; scans not sens because not enough blastic activity in the lesions; MRI used to evaluate cord compres-sion

Rx:

Therapeutic (Med Clin N Am 1992;76:371): Initial therapy: melphalan and prednisone (MP); little rationale for using interferon as initial therapy (Semin Oncol 1991;18:18); multiagent chemotherapy better for those w a poor prognosis (J Clin Oncol 1992; 10:334); maintenance therapy: interferon prolongs remission (Semin Oncol 1991;18:37; Nejm 1990;322:1430); resistant disease: vincristine, doxorubicin, dexamethasone, watch for toxicity (Ann IM 1986;105:8); high-dose therapy not recommended for the elderly

Supportive Therapy: Hyperviscosity: plasmapheresis; anemia: erythropoietin (Nejm 1990;322:1693; Blood 1996;87:2675), transfusions; hypercalcemia: biphosphonates; immunization w pneumovax recommended but frequently ineffective because of failure to induce antibodies

ONCOLOGY

LUNG CANCER

Am Fam Phys monograph 1995;191:26

Cause: 85%–90% from smoking; 15 yr must elapse for risk to approach that of nonsmokers; also from radon, nickel, chromium, asbestos

Epidem: Most common cause of death due to cancer; greatest prevalence in the 65-and-older group (Jama 1987;258:921); increasing incidence in women because of increased smoking in present cohorts of elderly (Radiol Clin N Am 1994;32:1; Cancer Pract 1995;3:13)

Crs: Elderly have more localized disease at dx than do middle-aged pts; more squamous cell carcinoma and less adenocarcinoma; small-cell lung cancer decreases; therefore, elderly have more resectable and, hence, curable lung cancer (Cancer 1987;60:1331)

90% of pts w recurrent lung cancer have distant metastases; most recurrences within 2 yr of primary lung cancer

Solitary nodule r/o secondary metastasis, carcinoid tumor, granu-

Table 7-2. Non-Small-Cell (Adenocarcinoma, Large-Cell, Squamous Cell) Lung Cancer

Stage	Treatment	Median Survival
Stage I (not involving entire lung, no node involvement or metastases)	Lobectomy	60 mo w small lesion, 27 mo w large lesion
Stage II (ipsilateral peribronchial or hilar lymph node involvement)	Lobectomy or pneumonectomy (right lung particularly high risk in elderly (Clin Sym 1993; 45:20); postop chemotherapy may be helpful (cisplatin-based)	17–20 mo
Stage IIIA (entire lung without involvement of the carina, ipsilateral metastases to mediastinal, and subcarinal lymph nodes)	Surgery plus chemotherapy, and radiotherapy (Nejm 1990;323:940)	8–11 mo
Stage IIIB (invading mediastinum, pleural effusion, contralateral lymph nodes)	—	—
Stage IV (distant metastases)	Radiation for pain, obstruction, hemoptysis	6 mo

loma, bronchiogenic cyst; dx of small-cell lung cancer in a non-smoker should raise the question of misdiagnosis of lymphoma

Lab: Sputum cytology—90% accurate, but not for individual histopathology; fiberoptic bronchoscopy well tolerated by elderly (Chest 1989;951043); hgb and hct; pleural effusion: thoracentesis w or w/o pleural biopsy

Xray: Chest film peripheral lesion needle bx or resection

CT: enlarged hilar nodes; bronchoscopy; if hilar nodes, obtain CT of liver, upper abdomen, brain, bone to determine metastasis; if mediastinal nodes enlarged, obtain mediastinoscopy to determine resectability

Rx:

Therapeutic: Tables 7-2, 7-3

Team Management: Determine if pt will tolerate surgery: FEV_1 >2.5: will tolerate pneumonectomy; FEV_1 >1.1: will tolerate

Table 7-3. Small-Cell Lung Cancer

	Treatment	Survival
Limited	Radiation primary tumor, and mediastinum +/− cranial irradiation (dementia can occur); if aggressive chemo rx cannot be tolerated, try VP-16 (Ger Rev Syllabus 1996; p. 327)	14–18 mo, 15%–25% survive 2 yr and considered cured, high association w second primary cancers (Nejm 1992;327:1618)
Extensive	Oral etoposide (Semin Oncol 1990;17:49)	9–11 mo

lobectomy; do elderly have higher operative mortality rates? yes (J Thorac Cardiovasc Surg 1083;86:654), no (Jama 1987;258: 927); function most predictive of postop outcome; poor prognostic signs include advanced disease, weight loss, nonambulatory for non-small-cell lung cancer; and increased age, elevated LDH, alkaline phosphatase, hyponatremia for small-cell lung cancer

Routine f/u after primary lung cancer treatment: history and physical examination (H+P) (pulmonary, abdominal, neurologic sx; cervical, axillary, and scalene lymph nodes; edema of face and neck), and chest xray q 4 mo for 2 yr, then q 6 mo–1 yr

BREAST CANCER

Am Fam Phys monograph 1995;191; Surg Clin N Am 1994;74:145

Cause: Risk factors: breast cancer in 1st-degree relative (Jama 1993;270: 1563), age >30 at birth of first child, late menopause, benign breast disease, heavy radiation exposure, conjugated estrogens, obesity, decreased bone mineral density (Jama 1996;276:1404), moderate alcohol use; 1–2× that of healthy age-matched controls (Nejm 1992;327:319); dysplasia in 5%–10% of benign bx specimens = 4× risk; hereditary in 5%, usually younger women

Epidem: Most common cancer in women; incidence in women <50 has declined by 13%, but increased in women >50 by 7%; half of breast cancers occur in women >65 yr old

Pathophys: Elderly women more likely to have well-differentiated cancer; both estrogen and progesterone receptors present in 60%–70% of elderly pts; biologically less aggressive than in younger women

Si: Masses more likely malignant in elderly women

Crs: Overall course more benign, more at risk for subsequent colon cancer (Am J Gastroentcrol 1994;84:835)

Compl: Elderly more at risk for emergency complications, eg, hypercalcemia, spinal cord compression, symptomatic brain metastasis

Lab: CEA, CA-15-3

Xray: May not see palpable lesion on mammography 20% of the time; palpable lesion in postmenopausal women requires bx; bone scans, CT of abdomen, pelvis, chest, and brain not called for in asx pts w normal physical exam findings

Rx:

Preventive: See p 42

Therapeutic: Surgical treatment w curative intent similar to that adopted in younger pts is appropriate for women >70 (J Am Soc Ger 1996;44:390)

Contraindications for breast-conserving surgery: tumor mass >5 cm, large breast size, subareolar lesion

Cancers >4 cm, preoperative chemotherapy results in substantial tumor shrinkage, allowing for breast-conserving surgery (J Natl Cancer Inst 1991;82:1539)

Excision alone ("lumpectomy") for tumors <1 cm

Postoperative adjuvant radiation therapy recommended for extensive cancers, eg, >4 pos lymph nodes; ER-pos more likely to benefit from tamoxifen (Eur J Surg Oncol 1994;20:207)

Frail pts w advanced localized lesions respond to tamoxifen (Jama 1996;275:1349) w 40%–70% tumor shrinkage, but long-term survival unchanged (Arch Surg 1984;1:548); tamoxifen well tolerated: decreases bone loss, increases HDL levels, increases risk of DVT, endometrial cancer, visual loss

Megestrol acetate (Megace), Anastrozole fewer side effects (Med Let Drugs Ther 1996;38:62); decrease recurrence rate w tamoxifen (Br J Cancer 1988;57:612)

Routine f/u of asx pts after primary breast cancer treatment: H+P (skin, chest, breast, abdominal exam) (Am J Clin Oncol 1988;11:451) q 3 mo × 2 yr, then q 6 mo × 3 yr, then annually after 5 yr; breast self exam q mo for life; mammography q 6 mo × 2 yr, then annually

Adjuvant chemotherapy survival benefit for healthy elderly women 70 yr old (Jama 1992;268:57); responses last 6–12 mo; most cytotoxic drugs metabolized in the liver; major liver dysfunction required to alter metabolism of these drugs; myelosuppression more common in the elderly; psychosocial adjustments to chemotherapy better in the elderly than in the younger population (Hlth Serv Res 1986;20:961)

Metastatic breast cancer: median survival 2 yr; palliative therapy for bone, skin, lymph nodes, pleural and pulmonary metastases; soft tissue and bone metastases will respond to hormonal therapy if they have responded before, eg, progestins, aromatase inhibitors, estrogens

COLORECTAL CANCER

Cause:

Epidem: Accounts for 14% of cancers in men and women; 3rd leading cause of cancer death after lung and breast; incidence 4–5× higher in people >65 yr old; two-thirds of colon cancers occur in people >65 yr

Pathophys: Minimum of 5 yr for adenomatous polyp to become malignant; if polyp >2 cm, 40% chance of being malignant; pts w cancers confined to mucosal layers, Dukes stage A (just mucosal involvement) have 80%–90% 5-yr survival; Dukes B (through bowel wall but no lymph node involvement), 60% 5-yr survival; Dukes stage C (involving lymph nodes), 40% 5-yr survival; Dukes stage D (metastatic), 5% 5-yr survival

Sx: Right-sided: anemia, abdominal discomfort; left-sided: hematochezia, pencil-thin stools, obstruction

Crs: 5-yr survival for overall colon cancer population is 57% and somewhat worse in geriatric age groups (CA 1992;42:9)

Colon cancer recurrence: most likely if tumor penetrated through colon wall; w poorly differentiated histology; presence of obstruction; elevated CEA; increased number of pos lymph nodes; rate of recurrence: 1st yr 50%, 2nd yr 20%, 90% by 4 yr, rare after 5 yr; 10% have second primary approximately 11 yr after initial colon cancer; pattern of recurrence: regional lymph nodes, then hematogenous spread to liver; 8% recurrence at site of original surgical anastomosis; local recurrence 25%–40%, liver 40%, abdominal peritoneal implants 12%–28%; metastasis usually concurrently 10%; solitary lung nodule has 50% chance metastasis and 50% chance of being primary lung cancer—therefore, need tissue dx; sx of recurrence: abdominal or pelvic pain, lower gi bleeding, change in bowel habits, weight loss, cough, bone pain; associated cancers: breast, ovarian, endometrial (Prim Care 1992;19:607); CEA elevation associated w tumor recurrence in 85%–90% of pts and may precede sx by 3–8 mo (Surg Clin N Am 1993;73:85)

Lab: CEA good to follow postop for recurrence; false-pos: smoking, liver disease, PUD, pancreatitis, diverticulitis, inflammatory bowel disease

Rx:

Preventive: 10-yr regular aspirin use in doses similar to those recommended for prevention of cardiovascular disease substantially reduces risk of colon cancer (Nejm 1995;333:609)

Therapeutic: Surgical excision only potentially curable intervention; rectal cancer—local resection w "pull-through" procedure to avoid colostomy, use transrectal US to determine depth of lesion and nodular metastasis; rx up to 3 solitary liver nodules w resection

Continuous infusion 5-fluorouracil—adjuvant therapy as effective w modulating agents, eg, leucovorin

IL-2 adjuvant rx

Monoclonal antibodies

Routine f/u: H+P, LFTs, stool guaiac for 2 yr q 3–6 mo, then for 2 yr q 6–12 mo, and after yr 4 annually; CEA q 2 mo for 2 yr, then q 4 mo for the next 2 yr, then annually after that; colonoscopy after surgical resection and 1 yr after that, then q 3 yr; chest film q 6–12 mo for 2 yr, then annually (Jama 1989;261:584)

Team Management: For hospice

- Bowel obstruction oncologic emergency: preventive: liquid or soft diet, stool softeners, antiemetics (metoclopramide); active conventional "conservative" iv fluids, antiemetics, vasogastric suction may resolve; if death imminent continue symptomatic rx only with pain relief and antiemetics; surgical treatment justified only in pt with >2–3 mo to live given high morbidity

- Obstructive uropathy common, may present with retention, dysuria, nocturia, frequency, decreased stream, etc.; treated with indwelling catheter or surgery
- Widespread pelvic metastases can cause difficult-to-manage neuropathic pain

PROSTATE CANCER

Sci Am Med 1995;12:IXA; Am Fam Phys monograph 1995;191:29

Cause: Hormonal, familial (Prostate 1990;17:337), oncogenic viruses, environmental, not associated w BPH (Lancet 1974;2:115), vasectomy (Cancer Causes Control 1991;2:113)

Epidem: 50%–70% of men >70 yr old have histologic evidence of prostate cancer on autopsy and <3% of them die from prostate cancer; nevertheless prostate cancer is the 2nd most common cause of cancer death in men; as much as 50% of cancers are clinically advanced at the time of discovery; well-differentiated cancer is least likely to spread (10-yr cancer-specific death rate <10%); most are moderate grade (10-yr cancer-specific death rate 10%–20%–Nejm 1994;330:242); poorly differentiated (10-yr cancer-specific death rate 30%–60%)

Incidence 0.8/100 000 in Asians and 100.2/100 000 in black Americans (Ann IM 1994;120:698); prostate is the most common malignancy in black American males and the 2nd leading cause of cancer death among black American men (CA 1992;42:7)

Men w father or brother w prostate cancer before age 65 yr have a 3–5× risk of developing prostate cancer; if they have 2 relatives who developed it before age 65 yr they have 5–8× risk

Pathophys: 95% adenocarcinoma; remainder are squamous, transitional, sarcomas; adenocarcinoma arises in the peripheral portion of the gland, while BPH arises from the periurethral area

Crs: PSA > 20 ng/mL or poorly differentiated, greater likelihood disease not confined to prostate; clinical pattern of recurrence: local pelvic progression; lymph nodes (obturator, illiac, para-aortic); bony metastases to pelvis, spine, and proximal femur; lung, liver, adrenal gland, supraclavicular nodes, brain

Lab: Age 60–69 yr: nl PSA range 0.0–4.5 ng/mL; 70–79 yr: nl PSA range 0.0–6.5 ng/mL; U.S. Task Force (1996) not recommend screening w PSA because finding prostate cancer early does not decrease mortality; one-third cancers missed w this screening test; false-pos as high as 60%; PSA density >0.15, more likely cancer and not BPH (Mayo Clin Proc 1994;69:59); PSA velocity >0.8 ng/yr more likely to be cancer (Mayo Clin Proc 1994;69:69)

Xray: Extraperitoneal lymph node sampling via CT-directed needle bx to determine staging and therapy (J Endourol 1992;6:103); bone scan to work up bony metastases; chest film, CT of abdomen and pelvis

Rx:

> **Preventive:** Large percentage of men w prostate cancer will not die from it; rx causes morbidity; therefore weigh risks in older people whose life expectancy is limited by other diseases
>
> **Therapeutic:** Routine f/u after primary prostate cancer treatment:
>
> - H+P (sx of bladder outlet obstruction, pelvic, spine and long-bone pain, neurologic sx from vertebral collapse, sx of renal failure, fixation of prostate to pelvic wall) q 3 mo × 2 yr, q 6 mo × next 3 yr, and after that annually
> - PSA q 3mo × 2 yr, q 6 mo × next 3 yr, and annually after that; PSA should fall radically in 2–3 d after surgery; extremely anaplastic tumors are not differentiated enough to produce PSA, so may not be elevated if recurrent

Nerve-sparing radical surgery for moderately differentiated localized prostate cancer in 70 yr old instead of expectant management increased survival time by 6 mo (Jama 1993;269:2650) improved survival for patients w locally advanced prostate cancer rx w radiotherapy and gorserelin (Zoludex) 79% vs 62% 5 yr survival (Nejm 1997;337:295)

> **Team Management:** Pts make decisions based on sx previously experienced, eg, choose expectant management if experience dribbling and radical prostatectomy if cannot start stream (J Am Ger Soc 1996;44:934); should refer to literature-based decision making by pt education video (The PSA Decision: What You Need to Know, video–Foundation for Informed Medical Decision Making, Hanover NH, March 1994); pain due to bone metastases; megestrol acetate effective for hot flashes in 60% pts; pelvic complications: lower extremity edema from lymphadenopathy, urinary dysfunction and neurologic impairment; oncologic

emergencies: spinal cord compression, obstructive uropathy, SIADH, disseminated intravascular coagulation

OVARIAN CANCER

Reinke D, American Academy of Family Practice Board Review Course, Seattle, 5/30/95; CA 1995;42:69

Cause: 80% benign; epithelial: 60%, and 5-yr survival = 20%–50%; mucinous: 5 yr survival = 60%; stromal sex cord tumors of which 90% are benign, two-thirds occurring in postmenopausal women; metastatic from stomach, colon, breast, uterus

Epidem: 1/70 women; most common gynecologic cancer causing death in women; 4th most common cause of cancer death in women; mean age 55–61 yr; industrialized countries; w ovarian cancer have 4× risk breast cancer; w breast cancer have 2× the risk of ovarian cancer; risk factors: low parity, high-fat diet, sedentary lifestyle

Pathophys:

Sx: Nausea, dyspepsia, lower abdominal pain; constipation; early satiety w omental metastases, urinary frequency

Si: Ascites; progressive weakness; weight loss; ovarian mass (normal post-menopausal ovary = 2 × 1 × 0.5 cm or smaller)

Crs: 3 hereditary patterns: ovary alone, ovary w breast, ovary w colon; usually detected in advanced stages; mean survival with residual tumor >3 cm = 21 mo; <3 cm = 53 mo; 75% present stage III—5-yr survival rate 10%–30%; prognosis: better with young age, good functional status, bcp's, small postop residual tumor volume, low tumor grade, low tumor ploidy

Staging:

I = limited to ovary—5-yr survival = 90%

II = pelvic ext—5-yr survival up to 70%

III = intaperitoneal metastasis or pos nodes—5-yr survival = 25%

IV = distant to lung, liver, peritoneal implants occur rapidly— 5-yr survival = 10%

Lab: Tumor markers: CEA—up in 60% epithelial tumors; also pos in cirrhosis, COPD, inflammatory bowel disease, smoking; OC125— correlates w disease in 93% pts; also pos in endometriosis, miliary TB, 1% healthy persons

Xray:

Noninvasive: US: solid w papillary projections w involvement adjacent visceral, distinguish cyst from ascites, bx metastases; transvaginal US even more effective; CT: for masses >2 cm, metastases; chest film, IVP, cystoscopy, proctoscopy, BE, UGI if sx

Rx:

Therapeutic: Surgery: laparotomy discouraged—spill cells; debulk to leave <2 cm, giving 5-yr survival of 35%; under 5% if bulky tumor remains; bx diaphragm, paracolic gutters, pelvic peritoneum, para-aortic, pelvic nodes, infracolic omentum; TAH/BSOO, omentectomy; 20%–30% pts require large-bowel resection; 5% require bladder or ureteral resection; ovarian cancer is a surface peritoneal spreader—rarely need diaphragm, liver, spleen resection

First-line chemo rx = platinum based combination, response rate = 80%; complete clinical response = 50%; paclitaxel (taxol) single most active agent in ovarian and breast cancer but risk of anaphylaxis requires dexamethasone as well as H_1- and H_2-antagonist antihistamines, if creatinine clearance >45 µL/min and good performance status without comorbid disease—age not a factor (CA 1993;71:594); only small portion achieve surgical response documented by 2nd look; even then complete surgical responders progress; 2nd-line chemo rx = interferon; granulocyte colony-stimulating factor (G-CSF) to prevent neutropenia with chemo rx

TREATMENT OF CANCER IN THE ELDERLY—GENERAL

Clin Ger Med 1997;13:169; Med Let 1997;39;996

Therapeutic:
- Oldest old tolerate radiotherapy in full doses without serious complications (J Am Ger Soc 1995;43:793; Curr Probl Cancer 1993;17:145; CA 1993;72:594)
- Nausea and vomiting associated w terminal illness: dopamine antagonist such as phenothiazine; benzodiazepine, antihistamine for anxiety
- Antiemetics for chemotherapy: start w prochlorperazine (Compazine), promethazine (Phenergan); serotonin-reuptake antago-

nist, granisetron in combination with dexamethasone more effective than either alone (Nejm 1995;332:1); ondansetron (Zofran) 0.8 mg tid
- Cachexia: megestrol acetate to rx cachexia, inconsistent results w increasing lean body mass; dronabinol, anabolic androgenic steroid, psychostimulants to promote appetite—no systemic studies in frail elderly

>1 in 3 conscious dying pts have severe pain (Ann IM 1997;126:97); pain management: analgesic dose in a pt who has become tolerant to a narcotic is not lethal because pt also develops tolerance to the life-threatening side effects of respiratory depression (McCaffery M, Phoenix, AZ, 1997); World Health Guidelines for stepwise approach to cancer pain:
1. Acetaminophen, ASA, OTC NSAID as well as nonpharmacologic interventions (radiation, relaxation, psychotherapy)
2. Weak opiate (codeine)
3. Graduated dose of strong narcotic (morphine)
- Equianalgesic doses: morphine 10 mg im or sc = 30 mg po = meperidine (Demerol) 75 mg im = 300 mg po = acetaminophen–oxycodone HCl (Percocet) 2 mg po = codeine 200 mg po = fentanyl 0.1 mg im or iv (Prim Care 1992;19:793); may need up to 1800 mg po morphine sulfate (Nejm 1996;335:1124); bone metastasis: 4 mCi strontium chloride 89 iv q 3 mo; neuropathic: 150–300 mg mexiletine tid; formal pt education about pain helpful (CA 1994;74:2139); fentanyl patch 21.5 mg q 3 d
- Biofeedback, hypnosis, behavior modification for chronic pain (Ann IM 1980;93:588)
- Terminal hydration leads to untoward effects such as pulmonary edema (Cancer Nurs 1990;13:62)
- Hypercalcemia: iv saline and loop diuretics; pamidronate 60–90 mg iv over 4 h, repeat q 2 wk; or calcitonin 4 units/kg im or sc q 12 h; or plicamycin 25 μg/kg iv q 4–6 h (Drugs 1993;46:594)

Team Management:
- Ethical dilemmas in feeding the terminally ill (J Am Ger Soc 1984;32:237; 1984;32:525; Nejm 1988;318:25) (see p 254)
- Family meeting w dying pt (simple nonjudgmental listening)
1. Have pt tell the story of how he/she became ill and the course of the illness; the pt may ask spouse to tell the story but it is

important that the pt do so, regaining confidence and connection w the family this way

2. Have pt talk about his/her worries and fears; first, fears for the family
   a. Spouse—describe how met spouse, evaluate the marriage, voice disillusionments, resentments so they may be let go
   b. "Children"—speak to each, reframe crying not as "breaking down" but as "breaking through"; important for pt to realize that he/she does not have control over how the children will live the rest of their lives and that he/she must let this go; can now only simply give the "gift of love"; grandchildren may have separation and individuation issues (Kubler-Ross E, Children facing death, Presented at the 4th international seminar on terminal care, Montreal, Canada, 1982)
   c. "Self"—his/her worries for him/herself: suffering, loneliness, fear, loss of control

3. Concerning roots: have the pts recount stories about parents and siblings, unmourned deaths

4. Family tells of the pt: spouse evaluates marriage; secrets may emerge (alcohol, incest) not to inflame guilt but to keep secrets from being buried only to reappear in future generations (Murphy M, Hospice Conference, New York, 1992)

• Transportation for radiation rx

8. Cardiology

HYPERTENSION

Ger Rev Syllabus 1996; p. 219; NIH Publc No. 93-1088; Arch IM 1993;153:177; 1995;155:563

Cause:

Epidem: 50% of pts >65 yr old have chronic HT; diastolic BP rises until age 55, when it begins to level off; therefore the rise in isolated systolic BP accounts for the overall increase in age-related HT: 10% at age 70, and 20% at age 80 independent of race; elevated systolic BP is the single greatest risk for cardiovascular disease in persons older than 65; LVH in hypertensives may confer an increased risk for ventricular arrhythmias

Pathophys:

- Increased vascular resistance results from age-related decrease in elastic tissue as well as the development of atherosclerosis; also a decrease in vasodilatory response to β-adrenergic stimulation, while α-adrenergic response remains the same
- Renally secreted prostaglandins protect; renin/aldosterone/angiotensin worsen HT, although not a major cause in the development of HT in the elderly; basal and stimulated levels of renin and aldosterone decline with age; however, older pts respond well to smooth-muscle relaxants and ACE inhibitors
- Calcium and sodium intakes modulate BP via PTHs and the renin-angiotensin system (Ann IM 1987;107:919)
- "Salt-sensitive" HT depends on Na^+ and Cl^- together; BP decreases w Na citrate (Nejm 1987;317:1043)

Sx: Sudden onset or recalcitrant HT suggests secondary HT, particularly occlusive renovascular disease

Si: Systolic BP >160 mmHg more significant risk factor than diastolic BP >95 mmHg (NIH Publc No. 93-1088)

Pseudo-HT w rigid arteries that cannot be compressed by sphygmomanometer cuff, giving falsely high readings, but can still palpate radial pulse (Osler's sign)

Crs:

- Older pts w HT at higher risk for orthstatic hypotension; rx of systolic and diastolic HT up to age 85 yr (NNT − 1 = 75 in preventing death) (Lancet 1991;338:1281); LVH decreases over 6 mo and function improves in elderly rx'd with verapamil or atenolol (Nejm 1990;322:1350)
- Isolated moderate systolic HT also associated w increased cardiovascular risks of 1.5× (Nejm 1993;329:1912)

Rx of isolated systolic HT (>160) in elderly reduces CVAs by one-third (NNT − 5 = 33) (Jama 1991;265:3255), stroke mortality by 36%, and cardiac mortality by 25% (Ann IM 1994; 121:355), NNT − 5 = 18 to prevent MI/CVA (Jama 1994;272: 1932)

Cmplc: Hypertensive crisis; chronic renal failure; cardiovascular including LVH, which increases risk of MI, CVA, Vtach, death, and sudden death 3–4× more than HT alone (Nejm 1992;327:998; 1987; 317:787; Ann IM 1986;105:173)

Effects on lipids (Geriatrics 1995;50(3):13): diuretics increase total cholesterol and triglycerides; β-blockers increase triglycerides and decrease HDL; sympatholytics decrease total cholesterol and HDL; ACE inhibitors decrease triglycerides; calcium antagonists have no effect on lipids; α-blockers decrease total cholesterol, LDL, triglycerides, and increase HDL; vasodilators decrease total cholesterol, LDL, and increase HDL

R/o sleep apnea (30%) (Ann IM 1994;120:382; 1985;103:190), alcohol and other drug/medicine use, primary renal disease, renovascular causes, pheochromocytoma, Cushing's, Conn's syndrome (Nejm 1992;327:543)

Lab: Routine initial w/u: urine analysis, K⁺, BUN/creatinine, EKG (3%– 8% sens) or echocardiography (100% sens, ? specif) for LVH

Xray: For renovascular HT: renal scan before and after captopril 50 mg po shows decreased flow in affected kidney (90% sens and specif) (Ann IM 1992;117:845; Jama 1992;268:3353)

Rx:

Therapeutic (Ann IM 1994;121:35): See Table 8-1

- Nondrug regimens (BMJ 1994;309:436)
- Avoid or stop NSAIDs (Jama 1994;272:781; Ann IM 1994;121: 289)

Table 8-1. Recommendations for Selection of Initial Antihypertensive Drug for Patients with Various Coexisting Conditions[a]

Coexisting Condition	Diuretic	β-Blocker	Ace Inhibitor[b]	α₁-Blocker	Calcium Channel Blockers Nondihydropyridine	Dihydropyridine
Older age	++	+/–	+	+	+	+
Black race	++	+/–	+/–	+	++	++
Angina pectoris	+	++	+	+	++	++
Post myocardial infarction	+	++	+	+	++	–
Congestive heart failure with systolic dysfunction	++	–	++	+	–	–
Cerebrovascular disease	+	+	+	+/–	+	+
Renal disease						
Serum creatinine <220 μmol/L	++	+/–	++[c]	+	+	+
Serum creatinine ≥220 μmol/L	++[d]	+/–	–	+	+	+
Diabetes mellitus without nephropathy	+[c]	+/–[c]	+	+	+	+
Diabetes mellitus with nephropathy	+[c]	+/–[c]	++	+	+	+
Dyslipidemia	+[c]	+/–[c]	+	++	+	+
Prostatism	+	+	+	++	+	+
Migraine	+	++	+	+	++	++
Atrial fibrillation (with rapid ventricular rate)	+	++	+	+	++	++
Paroxysmal supraventricular tachycardia	+	++	+	+	++	+
Senile tremor	+	++	+	+	+	+

[a] Symbols used indicate the following: ++, preferred; +, suitable; +/–, usually not preferred; –, usually contraindicated.
[b] ACE indicates angiotensin-converting enzyme.
[c] Requires special monitoring.
[d] Loop diuretic preferred.
From Jama 1996;275:1580.

- Dyazide (hydrochlorothiazide 25 mg + triamterene 50 mg) avoids all the MRFIT mortality risks (Ann IM 1995;122:223; Nejm 1994;330:1852)
- Calcium channel blocker; second choice in elderly after diuretics (Arch IM 1991;151:1954), eg, diltiazem SR 60–180 mg bid, although some studies suggest produces more cognitive impairment than atenolol (Ann IM 1992;116:615); ? decrease or increase mortality controversy (J Am Ger Soc 1995;43:1309); black men do best with diltiazem: 85% success rate compared w 33% w captopril (1995;8:189), association of cancer w calcium channel blockers (Am J Hypertens 1996;9:695)
- Do not lower below 140/85 mmHg (Swedish trial in old persons w HT, STOP-HT: Lancet 1991;338:1281); Finnish cohort study: lowering BP 5 mmHg from 90 to 86 associated w decreased 5-yr survival (J Hypertens 1994;7:1183); when withdraw pts from chronic antihypertensives, 40% of pts require restarting them within 1 yr (J Intern Med 1994;235:581)
- Decrease systolic BP below 160 mmHg; older pts more sensitive to volume depletion and sympathetic inhibition, therefore more prone to hypotension; start w smaller doses of diuretics and β-blockers, and longer periods between doses, measure BP lying and standing; chlorthalidone 2.5 mg qd for isolated cystolic hypertension results in 80% risk reduction of CHF in patients w prior MI (Jama 1997;378:212)
- ACE inhibitor may best preserve renal function even w early renal failure, eg, enalapril 5 mg po qd-qid (NNT = 4) (BMJ 1994;309:833)
- Rx of HT crisis (Nejm 1990;323:1178; Med Let Drugs Ther 1989;31:32): nitroprusside drip or propranolol 1–3-mg bolus q 5–10 min iv best; nifedipine 10–20 mg sl with pinholed capsule; labetolol 20–80 mg over 20 sec up to 300 mg q 10 min iv; diazoxide 50–150 mg iv q 5 min with propranol 3 mg/h and/or diuretic; hydralazine 10–20 mg iv × 1; then, po nifedipine, clonidine, or captopril; all require extreme caution in use in elderly

CORONARY ARTERY DISEASE

Ger Rev Syllabus 1996; p. 222

ATHEROSCLEROSIS

Nejm 1996;344:1311; J Am Coll Cardiol 1995;25:1000 (women)

Cause: Cholesterol (Nejm 1981;304:65), smoking, HT, lack of estrogen (Ann IM 1976;85:447), genetic (especially in women); not increased by triglyceride elevations alone, although they are markers for other risk factors (Nejm 1993;328:1220)

Epidem: By age 70 yr, 15% of men and 9% of women have symptomatic CAD; 70%–80% of deaths among people >65 yr

Increased in diabetes, HT, obesity (Nejm 1990;322:882), homocystinuria (Jama 1992;268:877)

Low HDL predicts cardiac mortality in pts >70 yr old, elevated total cholesterol not associated w mortality in men but may be in women (Jama 1995;274:539)

Decreased in women who take postmenopausal estrogens (Nejm 1991;325:756)

Pathophys (Nejm 1992;326:242,310): Earliest change: lipid-laden cells or fatty streak in intimal layer of artery (Am Heart J 1994;128:1300)

Wall stress causes fibrous plaques which later infiltrate with cholesterol; impaired fibrinolysis may also play a role in genesis; IL-1, cytokines suggest immunologic mechanism (Basic Res Cardiol 1994;89:41); HDL protective because it stabilizes vasodilator prostaglandin I_2 (Circ 1994;90:1033); HT may induce endothelial dysfunction (Hypertension 1995;25:155); hemorrhage into plaque causes sudden occlusions

Sx: Claudication, angina, MI, sudden death, TIA/CVA, abdominal angina

Si: Renal HT; bruits, absent peripheral pulses; CVAs; retinal fundal vessel plaques

Crs: Reversible with rx? (Ann IM 1994;121:348)

Rx:

- Rx of elevated cholesterol (LDL $\geq$ 130 mg/dL, NH Med 1997; Supplement D:ID) if two other cardiac risk factors (Ger Rev Syllabus

1996; p. 84), which helps both by decreasing plaques and by preventing coronary artery spasm (Nejm 1995;332;481,488; Circ 1994;89:1329; 1994;90:1056; Lancet 1994;334:1383); reducing cholesterol may be hazardous (BMJ 1994;308:373)

- Exercise (Jama 1995;273:402) decreases hospitalizations (J Am Ger Soc 1996;44:113); maximum heart rate for men is 220 minus age and for women is 220 minus 0.6× (age) because maximal ionotropic and chronotropic response to catecholamine and sympathetic nervous system is markedly impaired
- ASA: 1 tab qod (Nejm 1992;327:175; 1989;321:129) or qd 75–325 mg (Med Let Drugs Ther 1995;37:14; Arch IM 1995;155:1386) after angina or MI
- Diet that produces LDL <100 induces plaque regression (Lancet 1994;344:1383); "Mediterranean diet" helps (Lancet 1994;343: 1454); Diet: <30% fat, <7% saturated fat, <200 mg chol/d, then HMG-CoA reductase inhibitor; nictotinic acid 1.5–3.0 g/d (lowers triglycerides, increases HDL) (Am Fam Phys 1997;55:2250); estrogen replacement decreases ASHD incidents in women by up to 50% (Jama 1995;273:199); alcohol at 2–3 drinks qd decreases mortality by 25% (Am J Pub Hlth 1993;83:805); perhaps vit E, an antioxidant, prevents LDL oxidation and decreases ASHD 40% (Nejm 1993;328:1444,1450; Am Heart J 1994;128:1333)
- Estrogen/progesterone reduces risk by 50% (Jama 1995;273: 199,240); perhaps medroxyprogesterone to increase HDL cholesterol in postmenopausal females (Nejm 1981;304:560); EDTA chelation of various heavy metals no help (Med Let Drugs Ther 1994; 36:48)
- Preop assessment of cardiac risks:
  Clinical variables: <6 mo s/p MI, advanced age, h/o angina, non Q-wave MI, DM, HT, ventricular ectopy requiring rx; asx pts w bradycardia or chronic bifascicular block do not need prophylactic pacing
  Preop angioplasty in pts w >3 clinical variables and dipyridamole thallium test that demonstrates either redistribution of EKG changes associated w dipyridamole infusion; if 1–2 clinical variables and pos thallium, risk of having cardiac event (unstable angina, MI, pulmonary edema, cardiac death) increased from 3.0% to 30% (Nejm 1996;344:1311)
  61% of MIs in 1st wk postop are silent

CARDIOLOGY

ANGINA

Mod Concepts Cardiovasc Dis 1988;57:19; Nejm 1984;310:1712; Am Fam Phys 1994;49:1459

Cause: Atherosclerotic heart disease; myopathic disorders; mitral valve prolapse; reduced vasodilator reserve in coronary arteries (Nejm 1993;328:1659,1706); mental stress is as good an inducer of angina as exercise (Nejm 1988;318:1005)

Epidem: Silent ischemia: coexistent w angina: potential benefit of β-blockers, calcium channel blockers, coronary revascularization (J Am Ger Soc 1996;44:83)

Pathophys: Spasm may occur even when there is no fixed lesion, unstable angina usually due to a platelet thrombus (Nejm 1992;326:287)

Sx: Onset with first exercise after rest; more frequently in unfamiliar settings; worse supine; relieved by TNG (r/o esophogeal spasm pain)

Si: S_4; mitral regurgitant murmur during pain

Crs: Prognosis depends on extent of coronary involvement evidenced by angiography, and LV function (Circ 1994;90:2645)

Cmplc: MI

R/o esophageal reflux (which can mimic exactly) (Ann IM 1992;117:824); PUD, biliary colic, pleurisy, pancreatitis, pulmonary infarct, pneumothorax (Geriatrics 1995;50(9):33); carbon monoxide induction if onset at home in winter (Nejm 1995;322:48)

Lab:

Chemistry: CPK-MB may elevate mildly

Noninvasive: ETT contraindicated in CHF, aortic stenosis, IHSS, unstable angina; can't interpret ST changes in face of LBBB, WPW, digoxin, LVH; submaximal test (<85% maximal pulse achieved)

Depressions go from 0.5 mm to >2 mm and start in first 3 min or last 8 or more min (Nejm 1979;301:230) and/or hypotension during ETT—scoring system predicts 5-yr survival and annual mortality (Nejm 1991;325:849)

Thallium scan at peak exercise and 2–4 hr later; a better predictor of long-term outcome than ETT or Holter (Ann IM 1990;113:575); dipyridamole (Persantin) used when pt cannot walk on treadmill

Echocardiogram w dobutamine stress (Am J Cardiol 1993;72:605); about same sens and specif as dipyridamole thallium

Rx:

- ASA 75–325 mg po qd prevents MIs
- Antianginal meds (Med Let Drugs Ther 1994;36:111)

    Nitrates to dilate, reduce spasms, increase collaterals, and decrease platelet adhesion; po, sl, buccal patch or paste; tolerance develops so avoid hs or 24-h rx

    β-Blockers decrease pulse, block action of sympathetic nervous system caused by mental stress (Circ 1994;89:762), lower BP, decrease platelet adhesion; avoid in Prinzmetal type because can increase spasm

    Calcium channel blockers dilate, reduce spasm

    Imipramine 50 mg po hs helps microvascular

- Surgical

    Angioplasty (Nejm 1994;331:1037,1044; 1994;330:981) preferred in severely symptomatic pt w 1-vessel or 2-vessel CAD and nl LV EF, w multiple medical problems, increased risk for stroke w CABG because of cerebrovascular disease or diffuse aortic disease, increased risk for developing postop cognitive dysfunction, or frail physical condition; but more complications than medical rx (Nejm 1992;326:10); angioplasty long term requires more antianginal med and surgical interventions than CABG (Nejm 1994; 331:1037)

    CABG increases survival significantly (Lancet 1994;344;563; Circ 1994;89:2015); preferred in high-risk symptomatic elderly (even age >80 yr–Ann IM 1990;113:423) w left main artery disease, in pts w significant 3-vessel disease with EF >30% (Nejm 1988; 319:332; 1987;316:981), in pts w significant 2-vessel disease, decreased LV EF, and proximal left anterior descending artery disease, in pts w clinical evidence of heart failure during ischemic episodes w ischemic but viable myocardium w few other medical problems, younger physiologic age, and in pts who are prepared for 3–4-mo convalescence; diabetic pts do better w CABG than angioplasty (Nejm 1996;335:1290)

- Of unstable angina: ASA 75–325 po qd (Nejm 1992;327:175) in men (Nejm 1983;309:396); heparin alone or better with TNG (Nejm 1988;319:1105); thrombolysis no help (Circ 1994;89: 1545)
- Of silent ischemia: angioplasty (J Am Coll Cardiol 1994;24:11), atenolol (Circ 1994;90:762)

MYOCARDIAL INFARCTION

Am J Med 1992;43:315

Cause: Atherosclerotic (85%) including spasm; emboli (15%–Ann IM 1978;88:155)

Epidem: Increased incidence with h/o:

- Surgical menopause pts not placed on estrogen; but no sharp increase in natural menopause or BSOO pts put on estrogen (Nejm 1987;316:1105)
- Smoking increases risk 3×, but risk decreases to normal over 2 yr after stopping (Nejm 1985;313:1511); increases risk 5× if >1 ppd, 2× if 1–4 cigarettes qd in women (Nejm 1987;317:1303)
- Elevations of total and/or LDL cholesterol (often with cholecystitis hx) (Nejm 1981;304:1396)
- Diabetic, hypertensive women at higher risk for MI (F = 23%, M = 15%), and mortality rate as high as 46%
- HT

Decreased incidence with exercise, >6 METS >2 h/wk divided 3–4×/wk (Nejm 1994;330;1549); 2–3 alcoholic drinks qd (Nejm 1993;329:1829; Ann IM 1991;114:967)

Elderly undertreated and lidocaine overused (Arch IM 1996;156:805)

Pathophys: Platelet aggregations and thrombi (Nejm 1990;322:1549); early morning increase in catecholamine-induced platelet aggregation and decrease in plasminogen activator inhibitor type 1 contribute to thrombogenesis (J Am Coll Cardiol 1993;22:1228)

Sx: Chest pain, substernal, in "distribution of a tree," worse supine; diaphoresis, dyspnea; associated with heavy exertion

CNS sx, especially confusion, are the presenting sx in 50% of pts over 60 yr old; silent MI more common in the elderly, 15%–20% of MIs, DM often the cause

Si: Elderly may present w flash pulmonary edema, arrhythmia, sudden drop in BP, delirium, sudden weakness; in pts who have dementia or language barrier any pain in torso could be MI

Pericardial rub on day 2+, usually without ST changes (Nejm 1984;311:1211); S_4 gallop; fever <103°; transient S_2 paradoxical split (Geriatrics 1995;50(10):2)

RV infarct syndrome (Nejm 1994;330:1211): acute inferior MI, high CVP with low PAPs and PCWPs

Rectal exam important for guaiac and detection of BPH so do not omit on admission physical

Crs: One-third are "silent" and unrecognized (Ann IM 1995;122:96); prognosis is similar for Q-wave and non-Q-wave infarcts although non-Q-wave MIs are followed by more infarcts and angina but are associated w less CHF (Jama 1992;268:1545); TIMI III registry: most severe CAD, least likely to get angiography and most likely to have the most adverse outcomes from their disease both in hospital and at 6 wk (Jama 1996;275:1104)

Cmplc: Mortality 4× higher in elderly
- Shock (7.5%–Nejm 1991;325:1117)
- Arrhythmias
- Rupture of septal wall more frequent in elderly than younger pts
- Pericardial tamponade (r/o RV infarct)
- Aneurysm, occurs in 40% with anterior MI, develops in first 48 h, leads to emboli, CHF, and PVCs
- Mural thrombi without aneurysm in 11% of anterior MIs, 2% of others (J Am Coll Cardiol 1993;22:1004)
- Dressler's syndrome
- Papillary muscle rupture causes CHF
- Heart block (Mod Concepts Cardiovasc Dis 1976;45:129) occurs in 5% of inferior MIs, 3% of anterior MIs, and in 100% with anterior MI plus RBBB causing a 75% mortality
- Excessive adrenergic tone: analgesia and sedation appropriate, β-blockers should be considered (American Heart Journal 1994;9:1)
- Atrial flutter: if electrical cardioversion unsuccessful, use procaine amide
- CHF: rx systolic dysfunction with dobutamine for pos ionotropic effect

Lab:

Chemistry: Enzymes (Ann IM 1986;105:221):

Total CPK and/or fractions up in 12 h, peak at 2 d, last 4 d; CPK-MB rise during 1st 6 h after onset of pain has 95% sens and specif and may be used for early r/o MI in ER (Nejm 1994;331:561,607); total CPK correlates with MI size, but may not be as elevated in the elderly (Mayo Clin Proc 1996;71:184)

LDH and fractions (isoenzymes 4 and 5) increased; r/o renal and red cell source

Table 8-2. EKG Changes in MRT

Area	Leads	Findings	Artery
Anterior	V_3, V_4	Q, ST elevation, T inversion	Left anterior descending
Anterior septal	V_1, V_2	Q, ST elevation, T inversion	"Watershed"
Anterior lateral	V_4–V_6	Q, ST elevation, T inversion	"Watershed"
Lateral	I, aVL, V_5, V_6	Q, ST elevation, T inversion	L coronary
Inferior	II, III, aVF	Q, ST elevation, T inversion	R coronary
Posterior	V_1, V_2	Tall broad R, ST depression, tall T	Associated w inferior
RV	V_1, V_2	ST elevation	Associated w inferior

AST (SGOT) up in 24 h, peaks at 2–4 d, lasts up to 7 d

Cardiac troponin I elevation is specific to myocardium, useful perioperatively when surgery may increase CPK (Nejm 1994; 330:670)

EKG (Table 8-2): non-Q-wave MI more common in the elderly (Mayo Clin Proc 1996;71:184), T inversions (r/o acute cholecystitis–Ann IM 1992;116:218); in RV infarct, these changes are present in $V_{3-6}R$, especially V_4R w 80+% sens and specif (Nejm 1993; 328:981); new RBBB indicates occlusion of anterior descending proximal to 1st septal branch (Nejm 1993;328:1036)

ETT: if angina or CHF in the hospital, do a mini-ETT on therapy, to 5 METS or 70% predicted pulse before hospital discharge (Nejm 1979;301:341); thallium enhances prognosis (85% sens and specif–Ann IM 1990;113:684,703); if asx, full ETT with or without thallium at 2–3 wk predicts 5-yr survival (Ann IM 1987;106: 793); in elderly w arthritis, COPD, may not be able to accomplish; may need dipyridamole thallium study

>10 PVCs/h associated with a 10+% 1-yr mortality (Nejm 1983; 309:331)

Noninvasive:

• Ventriculogram with technetium scan; if <40% EF, 1-yr mortality climbs steeply from 5% (Nejm 1983;309:331; 1992;327: 669); LV EF not as accurate a predictor of mortality in women who have experienced previous cardiac arrest when compared w similar men; such women more likely to die independent of LV EF size (Circ 1996;93:1170)

- Dipyridamole myocardial perfusion imaging defects have significant association w risk factors for cardiac death or MI
- Angiography indications: CHF, LV dysfunction (EF <50%); high-risk noninvasive test results; persistent sx, failure of medical treatment; previous angioplasty, CABG, or MI; malignant ventricular arrhythmia; contraindications: very elderly, significant risk of bleeding, coexisting medical problems, eg, liver disease, terminal condition

Rx:

- Prophylactic interventions: ASA (see coronary artery disease, p 179); stopping smoking decreases risk to baseline in 3 yr (Nejm 1990;322:213); lowering cholesterol helps (meta-analysis–Nejm 1990;323:1112), as does American Heart Association diet (BMJ 1992;304:1015); β-blockers help older post-MI pt (J Am Ger Soc 1995;43:751; Am J Cardiol 1994;4:674), adverse outcome of underuse of β-blockers in elderly survivors of MI (Jama 1997; 227:115); diltiazem for non-Q-wave MI (60–90 mg po qid); captopril 50 mg tid, if ETT is impaired to <40% (Ann IM 1994; 121:750; Nejm 1992;327:669) or acutely × 6 wk for all ? (Lancet 1994;343:1115) or at least for anterior MI (Nejm 1995;332: 80)
- Of acute MI: 60%–70% of coronary deaths before arrival at hospital; prehospital thrombolysis (Am Heart J 1992;123:181); aggressive rx of acute MI w angiography, angioplasty, and CABG of minimal benefit (Jama 1994;272:859 891; J Am Coll Cardiol 1995;25:47A) vs CABG beneficial (J Am Coll Cardiol 1994;24:425)
- Coronary care unit (CCU) rx: oxygen only when objective evidence of desaturation (AHCPR Publc No. 94-0602, 1994); ASA 325 mg po stat
- β-Blocker rx (metoprolol 5 mg iv q 5 min × 3, then 50 mg po bid × 1 d, then 100 mg bid or atenolol 50–100 mg po qd) if no contraindications helps prevent recurrent MIs (Circ 1994;90: 762); mortality reduction 40% in elderly (Am J Med 1992;93: 315)

- TNG rx (iv if volume ok) goal to decrease systolic BP by 10%; excessive reduction in BP may result in extension of infarct (Mayo Clin Proc 1996;71:184)
- Thrombolytics: several studies support the efficacy in pts >65 yr (ISIS-2, GISSI, ASSET, AIMS) but age distribution skewed in these studies (<20% in pts >75 yr old) (J Am Ger Soc 1994;42:127); contraindications: active internal bleeding, aortic dissection within 10 d, prolonged traumatic CPR, hemorrhagic CVA within last 2 mo, head trauma, intracranial neoplasia, retinopathy, persistent uncontrollable HT; relative contraindications: diabetic retinopathy, prolonged need for CPR; streptokinase preferred over TPA (more hemorrhagic strokes); ASA + thrombolytic rx better for survival (ISIS-2); ACE inhibitor (Jama 1995;273:1450; Nejm 1995;332:80) beginning 3 d after MI w EF <40%, if hypotensive stop; diltiazem for non-Q-wave MI if no LVH or CHF
- Rehab: depression in CCU s/p MI: 10%, 3–4-fold increase in mortality rate in 6 mo if persists; return to work part-time in 4–6 wk (Barker LR, Principles of ambulatory medicine, Williams & Wilkins, 1995:712); if can walk 100 m without angina or dyspnea, can do air travel 10 d after MI (Dardick K, Travel medicine—what the family physician should know, 16th Annual family practice review, St. Petersburg, FL, Bayfront Medical Center, 3/94); benefits; lifestyle changes, then thiazides, then β-blockers? (Jama 1994;272:842; Hypertension 1994;23:275)

CONGESTIVE HEART FAILURE

Cause:
- Systolic: dilated ventricle (cardiomyopathy 10% >65 yr old, ischemia, infarction, HT, MR)
- Diastolic: LVH (CAD, HT, AS)

Epidem: 50%–60% = nl EF in elderly (Curr Probl Cardiol 1987;12:1); at autopsy, 50% pts with CHF did not have CAD (Mayo Clin Proc 1988;63:552); diastolic CHF in absence of CAD has low mortality

Pathophys:

- Systolic: hemodynamics: increased preload, afterload, heart rate, contractility; neurohormonal: increase in sympathetic tone, SVR; increased renin leads to increased angiotensin which leads to increased aldosterone which leads to increase in sodium retention; decreased atrial natriuretic hormone
- Diastolic: prolongation of ventricular relaxation, increased myocardial stiffness, increased end-diastolic pressure

Sx:

- Systolic: fatigue, sx of prerenal azotemia, cool skin, mental obtundation
- Diastolic: congestion, exercise intolerance (stiff ventricle)

Si: JVD more reliable than peripheral edema in the elderly; rales lower half of lung not always CHF; need echocardiography (Jama 1994; 271:1277); tachypnea; tachycardia

Crs: 28% mortality elderly men; 6-min walk test provides independent prognostic data in pts w LV dysfunction (Jama 1993;270:1702)

Lab:

Noninvasive:

- Systolic: EKG evidence of LV dysfunction, eg, Q waves; echocardiography
- Diastolic: echocardiography

Rx (Figure 8-1):

- Systolic: asx pts—9% mortality reduction w ACE rx (Nejm 1992; 237:685); prolonged bed rest dangerous; exercise helps—4h/wk 75% maximum heart rate in home walking program (Jama 1994; 272:1389; Ann IM 1996;124:1051); oxygen rx helps

Mild to mod—class I–II: diuretic (may need thiazide + loop, or potassium-sparing thiazide + loop; may even have to try metolazone + loop; if BUN is increased, then must curtail diuretic rx, but ACE inhibitors help all

Mod to severe, acute—class II–III (15% 1-yr survival): digoxin decreases hospitalizations but not mortality (Nejm 1997;336: 525); ACE inhibitors preferred (reduce afterload, enhance myocardial shortening, increase stroke volume–Nejm 1991;325:303); ACE inhibitors decrease mortality with LV dysfunction (Nejm 1992;327:669)

Severe—class IV (50% mortality): add ACE (Nejm1987;316:1429); if still dyspneic, add nitrate (up to 60 mg); if low cardiac output

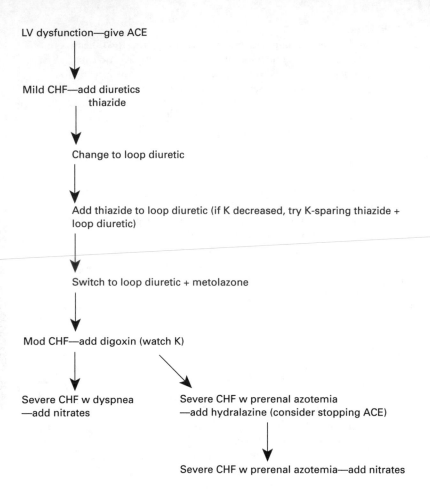

Figure 8-1. Flow chart for treating systolic congestive heart failure.

and prerenal azotemia, try hydralazine (up to 100 mg); if not tolerating ACE, ie, creatinine is high, try hydralazine and nitrate (V HeFT I–Nejm 1986;314:1547); hydralazine protects against tolerance of the hemodynamic effects of TNG, therefore use in combination in CHF (Cardiol 1995;26:1575); don't need to anticoagulate CHF pts (LV system dysfunction) if NSR (Jama 1994;272:1389)

- Diastolic: enhance effective ventricular filling; very sensitive to preload reduction, eg, nitrates, diuretics make worse
Rx HTN with ACE and it will decrease LVH by 15%; ACE promotes filling by reducing venous and arterial tone, regression LVH, attenuation coronary vasoconstriction; calcium channel, eg, verapamil (Nejm 1985;312:277)—not used for systolic failure because neg ionotrope
β-Blockers slow rate and promote ventricular filling

SYNCOPE

Ger Rev Syllabus 1996:p. 221; Sci Am Med 1995;1(4); Geriatrics 1995; 50(11):24

Cause:
- Yearly cardiac mortality—20%–30% syncope-associated: electrical, eg, Vtach, Afib, mechanical, eg, aortic stenosis in the setting of decreased preload or arrhythmia, pulmonary HT
- Yearly noncardiac mortality—5% syncope-associated: orthostatic hypotension (decreased baroreceptor sensitivity); positional; neuropathy usually present; Shy-Drager; meds: nitrates, diuretics, phenothiazines, tricyclics, antihypertensives; volume depletion; venous pooling; pts w HT more at risk for postprandial hypotension (Circ 1993;89:391); neurocardiac: vasovagal, cerebrovascular (arteriosclerotic vascular disease, carotid-basilar artery steal, subclavian steal) (J Cardiovasc Surg 1994;35:11); micturition; carotid sinus hypersensitivity R > L; psychiatric (panic): rare

Epidem: Annual incidence rate of 6% in the elderly

Sx: Cardiac (arrhythmic): premonitory symptoms are usually absent; vasovagal: nausea, fatigue, dizziness upon wakening; TIA: diplopia, dysphagia, confusion after episode

Si: Orthostatic BP from lying or sitting to standing after 5 min; carotid sinus massage only done when no carotid bruits—after 5 sec, produces 3 sec asystole or drop in systolic BP of 50 mmHg, then carotid sinus hypersensitivity likely etiology; aortic stenosis murmur (see p 192)

Cmplc: R/o seizures (bowel, bladder incontinence)

Lab:

Noninvasive:

- Cardiogenic (arrhythmic): monitor 24–48 h (Arch IM 1990;150: 1073), vs Holter monitoring not that helpful because complex ventricular arrhythmias recur despite treatment and 50% of pts without significant findings on Holter have recurrence of arrhythmias
- Electrophysiologic studies (EPSs) 3–4-yr mortality = 60% w abnormal EPS vs 15% w normal EPS; EF >40% correlates highly w neg EPS (Jama 1992;268:2553)
- Cardiogenic (nonarrhythmic): echocardiogram indicated to w/u aortic stenosis
- Cerebovascular: carotid US, cerebral angiography in pts who are good surgical candidates; CT not indicated unless focal findings or symptoms of neurologic disease
- Tilt table for pts without underlying heart disease to evoke vasovagal symptoms

Rx:

Therapeutic:

- Cardiac (see arrhythmias, pp 194, 195)
- Cardiac (nonarrhythmic): valve replacement for aortic stenosis
- Neurocardiogenic: avoid disopyramide, beta-blockers (Am J Med 1993;95:38)
- Orthostatic hypotension: elastic stockings, fludrocortisone 0.1 mg/d increasing to as much as 1.0 mg/d

Team Management: Education of physical activities/movements that bring on syncope, and careful discussion of drugs that cause syncope as side effects

VALVULAR DISEASE

Ger Rev Syllabus 1991, 1994, 1996
See Table 8-3

ARRHYTHMIAS

SUPRAVENTRICULAR TACHYARRHYTHMIAS

Ger Rev Syllabus 1996, p. 222; Am Fam Phys 1994;49:823,1805; 1994;
50:959; Nejm 1995;332:162; J Am Coll Cardiol 1994;23:916

Cause:
- Afib: associated w HT in 70% of pts; associated w mitral stenosis, atrial septal defect; also associated with hyperthyroidism or subclinical hyperthyroidism especially in the elderly (Nejm 1994;331:1252); toxic multinodular goiter present in 20% of the elderly with Afib associated w hyperthyroidism (Med Aud Dig 1983;30:18); alcoholic myocardiopathy; COPD; Aflut and multifocal atrial tachycardia often (60%) from pulmonary disease including pulmonary emboli
- Supraventricular arrythmias: hypokalemia, low serum magnesium; concomitant administration of digoxin and quinidine has 6.5% complication rate in older population

Pathophys: Afib: age-associated loss of sinoatrial node fibers, atrial myocardial fibers; amyloid deposition; atrial dilatation from decreased ventricular compliance; SVT re-entrant pathways

Sx: Polyuria, palpitations, faintness, neck pounding in AV re-entrant types but not accessory pathway SVT (Nejm 1992;327:772)

Crs: Afib: unfavorable markers for successful conversion: >1-yr duration or markedly dilated LA or recurrent after previous conversion

Cmplc: Elderly more dependent on atrial kick, therefore Afib may lead to CHF; 7-fold risk of stroke in nonrheumatic Afib and a 17% risk in mitral stenosis; post PAT T-wave inversions may last days to weeks (Nejm 1995;332:161); chronic Afib causes embolic CVA in 20% if recent CHF, chronic HT, or previous embolus (Ann IM 1992;116:1)

Table 8-3. Valvular Heart Disease

	Aortic Stenosis	Aortic Insufficiency	Mitral Stenosis	Mitral Regurgitation
Cause	Degenerative valve disease > rheumatic disease; associated w DM, hyperlipidemia; calcific AS age 50–60 yr (50% associated w CAD)	Rheumatic heart disease (mitral disease may also be present); cystic medial necrosis of the aortic root associated w aneurysm of the ascending aorta; HT and renal disease can lead to fenestrations of the valve	Rheumatic heart disease, 1/3 of mitral valve disease in the elderly	Rheumatic fever rare; CAD w papillary muscle dysfunction, ventricular dilatation, prolapse mitral valve, rupture chordae tendineae, CHF may be presenting sx
Patho-phys	Leaflet calcification in the elderly rather than fusion of the commissures as w younger pts	—	Commissural fusion fibrosis and calcification of leaflets and chordae	Calcium posterior cusp leaflets lifting them toward L atrium resulting in MR
Sx	Exertional chest pain, dyspnea, syncope; sedentary elderly: low-output state: weight loss, pleural effusions, hepatic and renal failure; Afib can lead to CHF in low-output state	CHF; more problems at rest than when they maintain exercise	Afib precipitates clinical deterioration	If dyspnea, orthopnea, edema, or fatigue present, valve replacement indicated; associated w Afib
Si	Low-output state: murmur not very loud; late peaking systolic ejection murmur as opposed to early peaking in AS; may be confused w MR; S₄ decreased carotid upstroke, associated AI murmur w calcific AS	W aortic root dilatation high-pitched blowing diastolic murmur heard best at the right rather than the left sternal border; wide pulse pressure; LVH	In older pts calcified leaflets less mobile, therefore first heart sound at apex is diminished, no opening snap; diastolic murmur heard best w bell at apex w pt in left lateral position; often associated murmur of mitral insufficiency	May be difficult to differentiate from AS in elderly because increased AP diameter results in diminished AS m. MR if not crescendo-decrescendo, and radiates axilla or left sternal border

Test	Doppler gradient >40; hemodynamic studies needed for low-output state; aortic area <0.75 cm² or peak systolic valve gradient of 70 mmHg	Pts where end-systolic dimension exceeds 5 cm² may be approaching LV dysfunction—indication for valve replacement before irreversible damage takes place	LAE on EKG; echo for severity	End-diastolic valve dimension >4.5 cm², refer cardiologist
Prognosis	W onset sx mortality rate = 30%–50%; aortic valve surgery (Circ 1993;88:17): encouraging results w human homographs; treat porcine and human homographs w warfarin for 3 mo at INR of 2–3, then D/C warfarin; mechanical heart valves: use warfarin long-term (INR at 2.5–3.5); ASA 160 mg/d may provide added protection; favorable results of CABG +/– valve replacement in pts >80 yr old (Cardicvasc Surg 1993;1:68); malfunction of aortic bioprosthesis if aortic diastolic murmur (Nejm 1996;335:407); surgery for asx pts if LVH dysfunction at rest, hypertensive hypertrophic cardicmyopathy, ventricular ectopy, pts may be denying their sx	Nifedipine delays need for valve replacement (Nejm 1994;331:689); replace valve w exercise intolerance and before LV dysfunction (Ann Thorac Surg 1992;53:191); presence of coronary disease worsens postcp outcome; may see associated rheumatic MS although less common in older people but when seen is more often accompanied by Afib than in younger pts; Afib worsens sx s of fatigue and CHF, and embolization may occur resulting in stroke	Anticoagulate if Afib present, valve replacement for progressive, severe sx's; malfunction of bioprosthesis if high-frequency holosystolic murmur (Nejm 1996;335:407); good outcome w valvotomy if class I or II (New York Heart Association)	If CAD present, operative mortality = 25% (Ann Thorac Surg 1993;55:333), then manage medically w diuresis, afterload reduction; Afib: rx w anticoagulation, ambolus less likely w MR than MS; good prognosis w valve repair of mitral valve prolapse

D/C = discontinue; LAE = left atrial enlargement.

Table 8-4.

PAT	Vtach
Regular even when aberrant and wide	—
QRS <0.14 sec	QRS >0.14 sec
axIs −30° to +120°	Left anterior descending

From Love J, talk, Augusta, ME, 9/85.

Lab:

> **Chemistry:** TSH
>
> **Noninvasive:** EKG; sick sinus syndrome is diagnosed by SVTs alternating w some heart block; suggested by P <90 after 1–2 mg atropine or asystole >3 sec after carotid sinus massage; supraventricular arrhythmias: normal QRS, regular tachycardia without visible P waves = AV nodal re-entrant arrhythmia: controlled w digoxin or verapamil (Table 8-4)

Multifocal atrial tachycardia: P > 100 and 3 or more different PR intervals and P-wave morphologies; looks superficially like Afib but digoxin won't help it

Rx:

> **Therapeutic:** Overall goal is ventricular rate control to protect cardiac output all but β-blockers may prolong or cause ventricular arrhythmias (Ann IM 1992;117:141); need to lower digoxin dose by one-half in the presence of quinidine to avoid digitalis toxicity
>
> • Afib (Nejm 1992;326:1264):
>
> *Acutely:* iv verapamil, diltiazem, β-blocker like esmolol, or digoxin to slow, conversion with digoxin alone is no better than placebo (Ann IM 1987;106:503) and rate is easily overridden by catechol/exercise stimulation (Ann IM 1991;114:573); if recalcitrant may need quinidine po (holds in NSR better but death rate is 3× placebo) (Circ 1990;82:1106) or procainamide or amiodarone (Ann IM 1992;116:1017) or clonidine (0.075 mg po, repeat in 2 h, decreases sympathetic tone) (Ann IM 1992;116:388); if LA size is <50 mm, use cardioversion (Mod Concepts Cardiovasc Dis 1989;58:61); if Afib lasts more than a few days, may want to anticoag-

ulate w warfarin before cardioversion (Nejm 1993;328: 750,803)

Indications for anticoagulation w Afib: ASA after TIA reduces recurrence of nonfatal stroke, MI, and vascular death by 20%–25% (BMJ 1994;308:1540); anticoagulate older persons w Afib w long-term warfarin at INR of 2–3; reduces annual risk of CVA from 7% to 1%–2% at any age (NNT – 1.5 = 25) (Circ 1991;84:527); annual bleeding risk ~2.5% (Ann IM 1992;116:6)

Nonvalvular Afib: ASA for pts <60 yr old, warfarin for pts 65–75 yr, ASA for pts >75 yr (Lancet 1994;343:687)

One-third in NH undertreated (Circ 1995;92:2178)

- PAT and Aflut: carotid sinus pressure; then, for PAT only, not Aflut—adenosine 6–12 mg iv, gone in 10 sec, potentiated by dipyridamole and carbamazepine, inhibited by theophyllines (Med Let Drugs Ther 1990;32:63); or verapamil 5–10 mg iv; perhaps propranolol iv 1–5 mg; then either digoxin + quinidine or electrical cardioversion with syncope; ok to do even if digoxin on board as long as levels therapeutic and not toxic and K^+ ok (Ann IM 1981;95:676)

- Multifocal atrial tachycardia: verapamil iv with pretreatment with iv $CaCl_2$ (Ann IM 1987;107:623) or po for chronic; Mg iv, especially if low; β-blockers if no COPD

BRADYARRHYTHMIAS AND HEART BLOCKS

Cause: ASHD, digoxin

Epidem: Idiopathic 3rd-degree heart block fairly common in the elderly

Sx:

1st-degree heart block usually causes no sx

2nd degree may cause dizziness or dyspnea

3rd degree may cause syncope, especially during standing

Si:

1st-degree heart block = PR >0.22 sec

2nd degree = some unconducted P waves

3rd degree = no relationship between P waves and QRS intervals

Sick sinus syndrome (sinoatrial node dysfunction due to CAD or sclerodegenerative process) presenting w chest pain, palpitations, or sinus pause, brady part of the bradycardia-tachycardia syndrome treated w permanent pacer

Crs: 5-yr mortality—50%; not significantly reduced by pacing, but pacer improves sx

Lab:

    Noninvasive: EKG; Holter monitor may still miss a majority of intermittent heart blocks (Nejm 1989;321:1703)

Rx: 2nd and 3rd degree: isoproterenol iv or sl, atropine iv, or external pacer until can get transvenous pacer; symptomatic pts w sinus pause >3 sec should be considered for pacemaker, as well as Mobitz type II block; pts w Mobitz type I should avoid digitalis, β-blockers, calcium channel blockers, and antidepressants

    Sick sinus syndrome: lower incidence of Afib w dual-chamber pacing (Lancet 1994;344:1523)

    Transvenous pacemaker: temporary first, then permanent, unless inferior MI, when block will usually reverse spontaneously; prophylactic pacers in bifascicular blocks only if 2 or more syncope episodes and even then questionable (Nejm 1982;307:137,180)

    Permanent pacemaker (RV–Nejm 1996;344:89; Mod Concepts Cardiovasc Dis 1991;60:31): dual-chamber types more expensive; use only when need atrial kick (Ann IM 1986;105:264)

    Pacer nomenclature:

Chamber Paced	Chamber Sensed	Sensing Mode of Response
Ventricle	Ventricle	Triggered
Atrium	Atrium	Inhibited
Dual	D	D
	0 (none)	0 (none)

Thus a VVI pacer paces the ventricle and senses ventricular beats by inhibiting the next paced beat; ventricular pacer cmplc: "pacer syndrome" (low cardiac output sx) (Ann IM 1985;103:420); tachyarrhythmias due to "endless loop" of PVCs causing a retrograde P, which is sensed causing a V pace causing a retrograde P, which is sensed, etc, can occur with any sensing pacer

DEEP VENOUS THROMBOSIS

Cause: Venous stasis from incompetent valves; increased hct leads to greater blood viscosity and clotting

Epidem: Occult cancers; extended sedentary periods (illness, travel); obesity; hip fracture; estrogen

Pathophys: Decreased levels of antithrombin III can lead to venous dilatation and stasis

Sx: None or calf pain; unilateral edema

Si: None or Homan's sign or increased calf diameter/tenderness/elevated skin temperature

Cmplc: Chronic postphlebitic syndrome: occurring after thrombosis involving destruction of the deep and communicating valves of the leg and obliteration of thrombosed veins; rarely painful; chronic edema (enlarged and hard leg because of trapped fluid from lymphedema due to scarring); hypopigmentation; stasis dermatitis; hyperemic ulcers; varicose veins; rx w 30-mmHg pressure stocking toe to knee; legs 3–4 inches above heart level at night if significant swelling persists; elevate legs intermittently, but ambulation should not be limited

Lab:

> **Noninvasive:** Duplex US: in pts w sx, better than IPG (Nejm 1993;329:1365); in high-risk asx pts only 38% sens (Lancet 1994;343·1142); in pts w sx's of recurrence it is difficult to distinguish on US up to 1 yr after initial DVT (Acta Radiol 1992; 33:297); use serial IPG if had normal IPG before; venograms may be indeterminate, therefore use degree of clinical suspicion in deciding anticoagulation (Geriatrics 1995;50:29)

Rx:

> **Prevention:** In hip replacement initiating low-molecular-weight heparin treatment (Nejm 1993;329;1370); 1 mo prior to elective surgery results in fewer DVTs (Nejm 1996;335:696)
>
> **Therapeutic:** Heparin iv × 5 d + warfarin started on day 1 (Nejm 1992;327:1485); continue warfarin × 6 mo (Nejm 1995; 332:1661); 1–2 mo only if transient specific cause; lifelong if recurrent idiopathic (Nejm 1995;332:1710); low-molecular-weight heparin as good as heparin for DVT (Arch IM 1995;155: 601)

ANTICOAGULATION

Anticoagulants

- ASA (Nejm 1994;330:1287) 75–325 mg po qd (Med Let Drugs Ther 1995;37:14) inhibits platelet stickiness; can be used safely w warfarin (Nejm 1993;329:530); adverse effects: gastric intolerance only at doses >30 mg qd (Ann IM 1994;120:184), asthma, increased bleeding time for 2 d, platelet dysfunction for 7–10 d; cheap

- Enoxaparin (Lovenox) 30 mg sc bid, low-molecular-weight heparin (Med Let Drugs Ther 1993;35:75) are clearly better with less bleeding (5%–Ann IM 1994;121:81) and better DVT/PE prevention over 6 d (Nejm 1992;326:975); $23/d as rx for DVT (Nejm 1996;334:677,682; 1996;335:1816); after 24° Lovenox may start warfarin and may discontinue heparin after ≥ 4 d and INR ≥2.0 for 2 consecutive days (Nejm 1996; 335:1821)

- Heparin: also inhibits activated prothrombin-platelet interaction; renal excretion, half-life = 105 min (Nejm 1991;324:1565); prophylactic regimen = 5000 units iv q 12 h; therapeutic regimen = 5000-unit load, then 1200 units iv/h; measuring q 6 h PTT until stable at 1.5–2.0× control

Prophylaxis of thromboembolism in surgical or orthopedic procedure where short term (<1 mo): recommended dosing: once-daily evening doses of 5.0–7.5 mg; lower doses should be used in elderly pts; during initiation of therapy, PT should be monitored daily, response to a given dose may not be accurately measured for up to 36 h, doses should not be changed for 3–5 d; 3 wk before treatment: hct, PT, APTT, and a platelet count; overlap prolonged PT 2–5 d with heparin as switch over (Nejm 1984;311:645) because it inhibits liver synthesis of factors X (3-d half-life), IX (1.25 d), VII (7 h), and II (4 d); INR of 2–3 for routine anticoagulation, 3.0–4.5 for artificial valves (ACP J Club 1994;120(suppl 2):52)

Preop and on warfarin: withhold 4 d prior to surgery and use heparin; discontinue antiplatelet rx 5 d prior to surgery and restart 48–72 h after surgery (Chest 1995;108:312S)

Warfarin (Coumadin) Protocol: INR <1.5, then increase total dose/wk by 10%; INR >3.4, then decrease total weekly dose by 10% after one dose is held; INR >6.0, then hold 1-d dose and give vit K 10 mg po and decrease dose by 20%; INR >10, then give vit K 5 mg iv and decrease dose by 50%

Adverse effects: bleeding, especially when given with probenecid or in renal failure; risk of serious bleeding = ~10%/yr in therapeutic range; correlates w higher PTs and 1st 3 mo of rx, not age or gender (Ann IM 1993;118:511); risk of intracranial bleed = ~2%/yr w PT 2× control, risk much higher if PT higher (Ann IM 1994; 120:897); blue toe syndrome (cholesterol emboli) rare complication (South Med J 1992;85:210; Surgery 1989;105:737)

Potentiated by foods and drugs (Ann IM 1994;121:676) that either displace from carrier protein or compete for degradation enzyme, including allopurinol (Nejm 1970;283:1484), amiodarone, antabuse, ASA, cimetidine (Ann IM 1979;90:993); or by decreased warfarin metabolism (cimetidine, erythromycin, tricyclics, Tm/S); vit K deficiency (inadequate diet, fat malabsorption, mineral oil, broad-spectrum antibiotics); unknown mechanisms: clofibrate, quinine, phenothiazines

Decreased w increased warfarin metabolism (barbiturates, carbamazepine); excess vit K (dietary supplements); impaired warfarin absorption (malabsorption syndromes, mineral oil, cholestyramine)

9. Pulmonology

CHRONIC OBSTRUCTIVE PULMONARY DISEASE

Geriatrics 1995;50(12):24; Ger Rev Sylllabus 1996; p. 278 (asthma, bronchitis, emphysema)

Cause: Smoking in overwhelming majority of pts; asthma may "reappear" late in life

Epidem: Asthma (increased bronchial and bronchiolar responsiveness to various stimuli resulting in airway narrowing): 1%–3% of new cases in the elderly, prevalence 3.8% in men and 7.1% in women, increased mortality in elderly

Pathophys: Normal changes in lung w aging: decreased elastic recoil resulting in collapsed airways during respiratory cycle, especially in lower part of lung leading to V/Q mismatch; decreased chest wall compliance, number of alveoli, vital capacity, maximum voluntary ventilation, FEV_1, maximum expiratory flow rate

Increase in residual volume and functional residual capacity; all of these changes accentuated by pulmonary disease

Limitation of expiratory flow, usually combination of emphysema and chronic bronchitis

Emphysema: destruction of air spaces distal to terminal bronchioles

Chronic bronchitis: daily production of sputum for 3 mo during 2 consecutive yr

Asthma: relatively few new cases

Sx: Fear of shortness of breath may lead to blunting of emotional response in interpersonal interactions (Heart Lung 1973;2:389)

Si: Final stages: cor pulmonale—barrel chest, prolongation of expiration, wheezing, pulmonary HT, elevated jugular venous pressure, pronounced pulmonic closure sound (P_2), hepatic congestion, peripheral edema, cyanosis

Asthma: indicators of acuity: difficulty walking 100 feet or more, speech fragmented by rapid breath, syncope, pulsus paradoxus >12 mmHg, inability to lie supine, accessory muscle use, respiratory rate >30; heart rate >120; FEV_1 or peak expiratory flow rate <30% predicted value

Cmplc: R/o lung cancer, CHF, GE reflux, recurrent aspiration, thromboembolic disease (pleuritic pain, hemoptysis, unexplained right-sided heart failure, hypoxemia), cough secondary to β-blockers, ACE inhibitors

Lab: Normal PaO_2 for patient >65 yr old = 80–85 mmHg (Eur Respir J 1994;7:856), PaO_2 decreased ≈ 3 mmHg/decade, 100 − (age/3) = PaO_2 for age; FEV_1/FVC <0.70; FEV_1 falls 30 mL/yr and 75–80 mL/yr in smokers

Asthma: reversible w bronchodilators: FEV_1 improves by 15% or 200 mL

Xray: Chronic bronchitis: increased bronchiolar markings, increased heart size; emphysema: elongated heart, hyperinflation of lungs, bullae

Rx:

Therapeutic:
- Bronchodilator therapy: symptomatic improvement, but does not change survival; 40% patients use metered-dose inhalers (MDIs) inappropriately, spacers help (correct use: National Asthma Education Program, National Heart, Lung, and Blood Institute, 1991:57); reasons for noncompliance include expense, memory lapse, denial, anxiety
- $β_2$-Adrenergic agonists most effective for acute episodes of asthma and prevention of exercise-induced asthma; long-acting $β_2$-adrenergic agonists prevent nocturnal asthma and should be prescribed only at regular intervals (never prn); elderly asthmatics have diminished receptor response and may not respond as well to β-adrenergic agonists (Geriatrics 1995;50(12):24); salmeterol not approved for COPD, just asthma (Nejm 1995;333:499)

Anticholinergic: ipratropium bromide best as chronic therapy in addition to $β_2$-adrenergic receptor agonists; not advantageous to use both in the acute setting (Ann Pharmacother 1994;28:1379), precipitates glaucoma if sprayed in eye

Corticosteroids: first-line therapy for asthma; loss of bone density if given systemically; rinsing mouth after inhaler avoids oral candidiasis, cataracts

Cromolyn anti-inflammatory blocks mast cell degranulation, 1–2

Table 9-1. Theophylline Levels

Increased Levels	Decreased Levels
Caffeine	β-Blockers
Erythromycin	Barbiturates
Clarithromycin (Biaxin)	Phenytoin
Ciprofloxacin (Cipro)	Rifampin
Pentoxifylline (Trental)	Felodipine (Plendil)
Cimetadine	High protein
Ranitidine (Zantac)	Low carbohydrate
Enoxacin (Penetrex)	Carbamazepine (Tegretol)
Disulfiram (Antabuse)	Smoking
Mexiletine (Mexitil)	
Ticlopidine (Ticlid)	
Estrogen/progestin	
Isoproterenol (Isuprel)	
Propranolol	
Flu shot	
Untreated hypothyroid, CHF	
Thiabendazole (Mintezol)	

puffs qid; nedocromil anti-inflammatory w sometimes unpleasant taste, nausea, vomiting, rhinitis occasionally

Theophyline (Chest 1995;107:206S) (Table 9-1): in older pts w emphysema may be of value initially for airflow obstruction that is irreversible; may reduce the work of breathing, augmenting diaphragmatic breathing and acting centrally to increase respiratory drive; may also work as a mild diuretic; high serum levels may be helpful to pts w asthma, but toxicity (nausea, cardiac arrhythmias, confusion, seizures) 17× more frequent in the elderly; therefore has limiting role in COPD (Nurs Home Pract 1995;3:17); erythromycin and cimetadine inhibit cytochrome P-450 metabolism of theophylline; liver disease and CHF reduce its clearance; decrease theophylline by 50% if giving ciprofloxacin at the same time; measure levels after 2–5 d of therapy; therapeutic trough = 5–15 μg/mL

O_2:PO_2 <55 mmHg or cor pulmonale or polycythemia w PO_2 <60 mmHg indication for long-term oxygen therapy at home; goal is to increase PO_2 >60 mmHg; after 1, 6, 12 mo, ABGs should be measured to determine ongoing need for and appropriate dose of oxygen; long-term oxygen therapy: increased survival, devices available (Nejm 1995;333:710)

Team Management:
- Avoid irritants: smoking, dust, air pollution, humidity; pts >65 yr gain 4 yr of life expectancy if they quit smoking; MAO inhibitors may help w the addiction, counteracting nicotine stimulation of dopamine release (Jama 1995;275:1217)
- For substantial sputum production: percussion and postural drainage given by a family member
- Severe dyspnea: conscious slowing of respirations, and purse-lipped breathing, relaxation techniques
- Arm movement exercise controversial
- Daily 15-min periods of exercise-induced hyperpnea increase ventilatory capacity in pts 65–75 yr old; 8-wk training program produces significant reduction in breathlessness (Geriatrics 1993;48:59); pulmonary rehabilitation program improves exercise capacity in older pts w COPD (Chest 1995;107:730)
- Nutrition: high ratio of fat to carbohydrate; fat metabolism generates the least amount of carbon dioxide, carbohydrates the most; very hot and cold foods stimulate coughing
- Psychosocial support; family education, eg, care and crisis
- Asthma: color-coded peak expiratory flow meters may make it easier for older pts to monitor asthma in outpatient setting (Am Fam Phys monograph 1995;2); stepwise approach to asthma management:
  1 Intermittent: prn inhaled β_2-agonist, less than once a week
  2. Mildly persistent: daily inhaled corticosteroid (200–500 μgm) w β_2-agonist prn less than once a week
  3. Moderately persistent: daily inhaled corticosteroid (800–2000) plus long-acting β_2-agonist plus prn β_2-agonist not to exceed 3–4×/d
  4. Severely persistent: inhaled corticosteroid (800–2000 μgm) plus long-acting β_2-agonist plus sustained-release theophylline plus prn β_2-agonist (National Institutes of Health Publc No. 95-3659, 1995)
- Always heed "subjective" responses to empiric rx trials as well as "objective" (eg, peak flow responses) since perception of breathlessness important to pt, reducing anxiety component

Preop Assessment: Only absolute indication for preop PFTs even in COPD pts is to measure lung volume before lung resection; consider local vs general anesthesia to avoid a 30%–50% fall in tidal volume; preop postural drainage w chest percussion to avoid complications postop; bronchial secretions increase for 6 wk after cessation of smoking, increasing risk for postop infection (Ger Rev Syllabus 1996; p. 65)

PULMONARY EMBOLUS

Cause:

Epidem: Very common; 15% of cancer patients will have one within 2 yr (Ann IM 1982;303:1509)

Pathophys: Thrombophlebitis causes thrombus migrating to lungs; recurrent small emboli more common than one big one; mostly thigh and pelvis veins (Ann IM 1981;94:439); no signs or sx's in 50%

Sx: Sudden, intermittent or chronic dyspnea; pleuritic chest pain w infarct; hemoptysis; fever; syncope w large emboli; common to have minimal sx's

Si: 33% pleural effusion of which 67% bloody (rbc >100 000/μL); unexplained arrhythmias; resistant heart failure

Crs: Resolves over 10–30 d (Nejm 1969;280:1194); 60% survival without rx, 90% w rx 3 d heparin; death in first 2 h

Cmplc: Chronic leg edema, chronic pulmonary HT

Lab: PO_2 <80 mmHg; A-a gradient: $PaO_2 = P_B - P_{H_2O} (FiO_2) - PaCO_2/R$, $P_B = 760$; $P_{H_2O} = 47$; $FiO_2 = 0.21$ for room air (RA) and 3.3/L; R = 0.8; PaO_2 for RA = $(150 - PCO_2)/0.8$

nl A-a = <10–15 mmHg and is abnormal if there is intrinsic lung problem

EKG: pRBBB $(S_1S_2S_3)$, right axis deviation 20%, $S_1Q_3T_3$

Xray: V/Q scan mismatch (PIO-PED–Jama 1990;262:2753); B-mode duplex US; arteriogram false-neg rate w 1%–5% complication rate, 1–4/1000 mortality rate

Rx:

Preventive: Mild to moderate alcohol consumption decreases risk of DVT and pulmonary embolus (J Am Ger Soc 1996;44:1030)

Therapeutic: Heparin 1.5–2.5× control × 5–10 d; overlap warfarin × 4–5 d and continue × 6 mo at INR 2–3 (Nejm 1995;332:166)

If major bleeding, stop heparin and allow anticoagulation effect to dissipate over few hours; if cannot tolerate warfarin long term, give heparin sc 10 000 units q 12 h; interruption of vena cava w filter for pts w persistent contraindication to anticoagulation; adverse effects include chronic leg edema, thrombus formation above the filter, recurrent embolization through collateral veins, perforation of vena cava, migration of filter

Aim of prophylaxis is to prolong quality of life; if pt terminally ill, eg, w cancer, anticoagulation may only prolong suffering

PULMONARY HYPERTENSION

Cause: LVH, valvular heart disease, COPD, chronic recurrent thrombo-embolic disease

Epidem: F > M

Pathophys: Excess platelet thromboxane A, deficient endothelial cell pros-taglandin (Nejm 1993;328:1732)

Sx: Dyspnea, chest pain, pedal edema, fatigue

Si: Right-sided S_3, pulmonary systolic and diastolic murmurs, tricuspid insufficiency, enlarged RV

Crs: If PA pressure <85 mmHg, then median survival time 2.8 yr

Lab: ABG: low PCO_2

Rx:

>   **Therapeutic:** Selective use of oxygen; low-dose diuretics; phlebot-omy for hct exceeding 50%; calcium channel blockers; warfarin anticoagulation (Nejm 1992;327:76)

PULMONOLOGY

10. Orthopedics/ Rheumatology

OSTEOPOROSIS

Nejm 1992;327:620; Bull Rheum Dis 1988;38(2):1; Ann IM 1995;123: 452

Cause: Primary:
- Type I: estrogen deficiency in postmenopausal women (Nejm 1984; 311:277) leading to trabecular bone loss
- Type II: slow bone loss starting at age 30 yr; 50% older females; 25% older males; trabecular and cortical bone loss

Secondary:
- Cushing's disease/syndrome (even 10 mg prednisone qd enough), including chronic oral steroid use in asthmatics (Nejm 1983;309: 265), RA (Ann IM 1993;119:963)
- Alcoholism
- Wintertime vit D deficiency (Jama 1995;274:1683)
- Anti–vit D meds like phenytoin, renal calcium leak (rx'd w thiazides); heparin
- Acromegaly, type I diabetes, scurvy, homocystinuria, hyperparathyroidism, hyperthyroidism
- Malabsorption
- Myeloma
- Bed rest—even short periods, particularly in elderly

Epidem: More in female smokers from changes in estrogen metabolism (Nejm 1994;330:387; 1985;313:973); less frequent in blacks and Polynesians because they start with higher adolescent bone densities (Nejm 1991;325:1597)

Pathophys: Simple estrogen deficiency postmenopausally (Nejm 1980; 303:1571)

Sx: Fractures usually of vertebrae, distal forearm bones, proximal femur; bone pain, especially vertebral

Si: Decreased height/kyphosis from vertebral compression fractures

Crs: Chronic, slowly progressive

Cmplc: Rib and vertebral fractures (Nejm 1983;309:265), hip fractures

Lab:

> **Chemistry:** PTH, serum and urine calcium to r/o hyperparathyroid and renal calcium leak in asx postmenopausal type (Spratt D, 1995); bone turnover markers: bone-specific alkaline phosphatase, osteocalcin (Geriatrics 1996;51:24); osteoclast-mediated N-telopeptide turnover in urine (Osteomark) (J Clin Endocrinol Metab 1995;80:3)

> **Xray:** Osteopenic bones and fractures; densitometry screening (controversial, much debated—Ann IM 1990;112:516; 1990;113:565; Nejm 1991:324:1105; 1987;316:212); might consider w pts indecisive re ERT or in high-risk pts (chronic steroid use, renal disease, hyperparathyroidism, Graves' disease, malabsorption); dual-energy xray absorptometry (DEXA) most precise and lowest cost (Am Fam Phys monograph 1996;1:1)

Rx:

- All rx is preventive or instituted to slow progression (Med Lct Drugs Ther 1992;34:101) (including progression of steroid-induced type) (Nejm 1993;329:1406); weight-bearing exercise (Ann IM 1988;108:824); smoking cessation, exercise (Ann IM 1992;116:716); posture and balance exercise (fall prevention)

- Calcium replacement therapy (Jama 1994;272:1942; Endocr Rev 1995;16:87—in men), as $CaCO_3$, 1–2 gm of elemental Ca^{2+}/d (milk has 300 mg Ca^{2+}/ cup; chewable Tums, 200 mg/tab; Oscal, 500 mg/tab) (Med Let Drugs Ther 1989;31:101); get to first 800 mg qd as calcium citrate (Citracal), higher cost but absorbed better, especially in achlorhydrics/elderly (Nejm 1985;313:70), then add $CaCO_3$ (Nejm 1990;323:878); substantial effect even without estrogen (Ann IM 1994;120:97), eg, 50% less loss/yr (Nejm 1993;328:460); calcium content in supplements and foods (Med Let Drugs Ther 1996;38:108)

- Vit D as 225–400 IU qd (400 IU in multivitamins, or as high as 600–800 IU) or calcitriol (D_3) 0.25 µg po bid markedly decreases fractures without producing stones by preventing increased PTH of winter at least (Nejm 1993;327:1637; 1992; 326:357; 1989;321:1777; Ann IM 1991;115:505); 400 IU × 2 yr preserves femoral neck bone density in women >70 yr (1995; 80:1052)

- ERT (decreases responsiveness of bone to PTH, preventing bone resorption) 0.625 mg decreases fracture rates by two-thirds (wrist, hip, other); even smaller estrogen doses (OB Gyn 1996;27:163) start soon after menopause and continue (Ann IM 1995;122:9) as late as age 75 yr; may also start as late as age 60 yr (Jama 1997; 277:543)
- Testosterone in men, especially if hypogonadism
- Bisphosphonates, eg, alendronate (Fosamax) (Nejm 1995;33:1437; Med Let Drugs Ther 1996;38:965; Am Fam Phys 1996;54:2053), 10 mg po qd clearly helps prevent progression over 3 yr, NNT − 3 = 10–30; prevents nonvertebral fx over 3 yrs (Jama 1997;277: 1159); analgesic effect (Bone Miner 1991;15:237); adverse effects: various gi sx, eg, esophagitis (Nejm 1996;335:1216); give w caution in pts w renal insufficiency; etidronate disodium (Didronel) 400 mg po qd − 14 d then 13 wk off in cycles (Nejm 1997;337:382); to avoid osteomalacia (Ger Rev Syllabus 1996:157); or pamidronate (Aredia) 150 mg po qd (Med Let Drugs Ther 1992;34:1); long-term value? when to stop?
- Calcitonin interferes w osteoclasts and inhibits bone resorption; 100 IU salmon calcitonin sc qd, which also relieves acute fracture pain, possibly via opiate effect (J Fam Pract 1992;35:93); 200 IU qd alternating nostrils (Med Let Drugs Ther 1996;38:965; Am J Med 1995; 98:452); nausea from calcitonin self-limited and <10% of patients discontinue med, other side effects include flushing, diarrhea, and pain at injection site; human calcitonin has more side effects than salmon calcitonin; recrudescence when therapy discontinued, even after a year of therapy
- Thiazides may help bone density and fracture rate (Ann IM 1993; 118:657,666; Nejm 1990;322:286); others report increased fracture rate (Nejm 1991;325:1)
- Sodium fluoride (NaF) in SR form 12 mo on, 2 mo off, appears to decrease fracture rate in spine when given w 400 mg calcium as citrate bid (Ann IM 1994;120:625,689), but is controversial (Ann IM 1995;123:401); 25 mg bid for no more than 4 yr (Med Let Drugs Ther 1996;38:965)

HIP FRACTURE

Nejm 1966;334:1519

Cause: Falls and osteoporosis

Epidem: 90% patients >50 yr old; rates lower in blacks, increased by thinness, maternal h/o hip fracture, alcohol use, CVA hx (Nejm 1994;330:1555), smoking (Nejm 1987;316:404), hyperthyroidism, visual impairment (Nejm 1991;324:1326), and drugs like long-acting benzodiazepines, tricyclics, and phenothiazines (Nejm 1987; 316:363) as well as other psychoactive drugs, especially in NHs (Nejm 1992;327:168); paradoxically also may be increased by restraints (Ann IM 1992;116:369); associated w being on feet <4 h/d, higher resting pulse rate (Nejm 1995;332:767)

Pathophys: Falls and fractures occur in the elderly because slow gait results in more sideway and backward falls on hips rather than on other body parts; diminished protective responses; less fat and muscle protection; diminished strength (J Gerontol 1989;44:M107)

- Subcapital fracture disrupts blood supply to femoral head; higher incidence nonunion and necrosis of femoral head
- Intertrochanteric fracture leaves blood supply to femoral head intact
- Subtrochanteric fracture does not interrupt blood supply to femoral head

Sx: H/o fall; hip pain (may be vague in the elderly)

Si: External rotation of the leg w shortening; pain w motion; persistent immobility in demented

Crs: 25% of fall-induced hip fractures result in death within 6 mo, 25% in subsequent functional dependence; 50% of pts are walking independently 1 yr after fracture (Am J Pub Hlth 1987;79:279); usually fatal unless repaired; prefracture mental status and physical functional level are best predictors of eventual outcome (J Am Ger Soc 1992;40:861); subcapital fractures make up one-third of hip fractures, w intertrochanteric and subtrochanteric making up the remaining two-thirds; r/o trochanteric bursitis, pubic ramus, acetabular fracture

Cmplc: After fracture, frequently develop in hospital (J Gen IM 1987;2: 78) confusion (49%), UTI (33%), arrhythmia (26%), pneumonia (19%), depression (15%), CHF (7%), DVT; femoral neck fractures: avascular necrosis in 20%, nonunion 30%; intertrochanteric: failure of fixation devices (tremendous muscle forces on bone) (Ger Rev Syllabus 1996; p. 245)

Xray: Fracture, often subtle, especially if impacted; best view: anteroposterior w internal rotation 15–20 degrees; repeat delayed films may be necessary

Rx:

> **Prevention:** W ERT; in elderly NH women, by 1.2 gm calcium + 800 IU vit D_3 (calcitriol) qd (Nejm 1992;327:1637) (see pp 207–208); w hip protectors in NH (Lancet 1993;341:11); thiazides? (Jama 1991;265:370); by avoiding use of slippery throw rugs in the home, restraints (Ann IM 1992;116:369)
>
> • Subcapital fracture: Austin-Moore prosthesis, early weight bearing; if nondisplaced: pin, weight bearing in 12 wk
> • Intertrochanteric fracture: screw w early ambulation
> • Subtrochanteric fracture: nail and rod, no weight bearing till healed

May need body cast to prevent dislocation in cognitively impaired individuals

Delay surgery if pt must be on anticoagulation; delay is associated w more postop risk (J Bone Joint Surg Am 1995;77:1551)

After surgery, consider heparin and/or warfarin DVT prophylaxis if pt not able to be up quickly, or at least compression stockings (Arch IM 1994;154:67); weight bearing in 1–2 d w Austin-Moore prosthesis, in 2–3 d w compression screw internal fixation, but not for 6–8 wk if pinned; can be discharged from hospital within 2–5 d

Loosening of prosthesis: groin pain w acetabular component and upper thigh pain w femoral component

Selected patients (advanced Alzheimer's, Parkinson's, CHF, CVA, near terminal illness) for no repair if high surgical risk or nearing end of ambulatory life; pain management often no worse or prolonged than w postop course

OSTEOARTHRITIS

Kippel J, Dieppe P, Practical rheumatology, Mosby, 1995; Jama 1996; 276:486

Cause: Aging: decreased proteoglycan aggregation, decreased resistance of cartilage to procollagen (Lancet 1989;1:924); obesity; postural defects (genu valgum/varum); excessive repetitive stress; crystalline deposit disease; previous inflammatory joint disease; hemochromatosis; Wilson's disease; acromegaly

Epidem: Uncommon <35 yr old, more common >65 yr old (30%–40% population >65 having sx); F/M = 1.5:1 (Arth Rheum 1987;30: 914)

Pathophys: Injury to articular cartilage leads to destruction of proteoglycan matrix, which in turn leads to cellular proliferation in attempted repair, release of enzymes with increased destruction of all cartilage elements, and proliferation of subchondral bone

Sx: Aching worse with activity; relieved by rest; morning stiffness; hip arthritis begins in groin and radiates to thigh, getting up from chair

Si: Late: joint crepitus; decreased range of motion, minimal soft tissue swelling + bony enlargement, minimal warmth or erythema; rare effusions; Bouchard's, Heberden's nodes; involvement of base of thumb; wrist not involved; knee > hip > spine, ankles, elbows, shoulders

Crs: Insidious onset; slowly progressive

Cmplc: Joint pain and instability; contractures, tendonitis, bursitis; r/o osteoporosis, malignancy, Paget's, osteomyelitis, reflex sympathetic dystrophy (RSD; precipitated by trauma, stroke, MI, skin of hand hyperesthetic, warm vasodilation proceeding to cold vasoconstriction w edema on dorsum of fingers; after 6 mo skin becomes atrophied, proceeding in 6 mo to diffuse osteopenia; 3-phase bone scan to make dx early in disease, rx w steroids, stellate ganglion block), neuropathy, parkinsonism, avascular necrosis of hip, trochanteric bursitis (lateral bone pain instead of groin/hip pain seen w arthritis, also still have range of motion and no radicular signs)

Of hand r/o hypertrophic pulmonary osteoarthropathy (clubbing fingers, swollen wrists); de Quervain's: pain in base of thumb elicited by gripping thumb under fingers and flexing wrist in ulnar direction, rx w splinting and steroid injection, surgery; Dupuytren's contracture: fibrous contraction of palmar fascia causing flexion of fingers, rx'd w stretching, steroid injection, and surgery

Of knee r/o anserine bursitis (medial aspect of knee), Baker's cyst, rx w steroid injection into joint helps because of direct communication w joint and cyst

Lab: Nl values (ESR, CRP nl); synovial fluid wbc <200/μL, protein <4 gm/dL, glucose ~ serum glucose

Xray:

Early: slight loss of cartilage thickness with narrowing of joint space

Middle: marginal osteophyte formation

Late: loss of joint space, sclerosis of subchondrial bone, subchondrial cysts, loose bodies, subluxation deformity

Hip films related more to sx than hand, knee films

Rx:

Therapeutic:
- Tylenol, ASA, NSAIDs (Nejm 1991;325:87) (see p 226); topical salicylates, other topicals worth trials (low risk); ice, cooling packs, corticosteroid injection; capsaicin cream not prn because takes several days to establish effects (see drugs, p 13)
- Joint irrigation through arthroscope
- Joint replacement good option in elderly without other medical problems; consider when major instability in weight-bearing joint, loose bodies in joint, intractable pain

Team Management:
- F/u frequently inadequate in clinical practice
- Exercise improves function (Jama 1997;277:25;1863), preserves range of motion and increases muscle strength and stability of joint; may reduce med requirements (Ann IM 1992;116:529); water exercises
- Emotional, social support; early education for long duration of disease
- Common splints: first carpometacarpal joint
- Assist knee and quad strength with appropriately fitted chairs and toilets
- Support proximal tarsal joint with lacing corset footwear
- Hallux valgus: rocker shoe helps reduce stress on joint
- Cervical pillow
- US deep heat increases tolerance, not cost-effective (Ann IM 1994;121:133), TENS for knee pain
- Assistive devices: jar holder, key holders
- Decrease weight (Ann IM 1992;116:535)

RHEUMATOID ARTHRITIS

Inflammatory rheumatic diseases in the elderly, UCLA Intensive geriatric review course, 1/96; J Am Ger Soc 1991;39:284

Cause: Humoral immune response (rheumatoid factor, IgM, IgG, or IgA complexed w antigens producing immune complexes w fixed complement) resulting in an inflammatory process; cellular immunity involving lymphocytes and macrophages; viral

Epidem: 20% new onset after age 60 yr—elderly-onset RA (EORA)

Pathophys:

Sx: Pain, inflammation small joints accompanied by constitutional sx's such as malaise, anorexia, weight loss; prolonged morning stiffness lasting >1 h

Si: Criteria for diagnosis: morning stiffness, arthritis of 3 or more joint areas, hand-joint arthritis, symmetric involvement, rheumatoid nodules, rheumatoid factor, radiologic features, at least 4 of which must be present for 6 mo

Extra-articular manifestations of RA occur more in young-onset RA (YORA): anemia, thrombocytosis, eosinophilia, Felty's syndrome, RA, splenomegaly, neutropenia, diffuse lymphadenopathy, osteoporosis, vasculitis, pericarditis w effusion, conduction abnormalities, valvular incompetence, Raynaud's phenomenon, pleuritis w effusion, interstitial fibrosis, bronchiolitis, entrapment syndromes (eg, carpal tunnel), atlanto-axial subluxation, monoarthritis multiplex, distal sensory abnormalities, autonomic changes, disuse atrophy, keratoconjunctivitis, scleritis, corneal ulceration, xerostomia, amyloidosis, cryoglobulinemia, hyperviscosity

Crs: 3 possibilities
- Few months of sx followed by complete remission
- Intermittent periods of active disease alternate w relative or complete remission
- Unrelenting progressive disease

Indicators of good prognosis: monoarticular, unilateral, proximal, more abrupt onset, brief duration of initial sx, male sex, absence of IgM and rheumatoid factor, absence of high ESR or CRP, no extra-articular involvement, no erosions on xray, milder course (50% chance remission vs 30% for YORA); only 6% w EORA have subcutaneous nodules vs 20% with YORA

Cmplc: Late articular complications: deformities of knees and hips result in decreased ambulation; subluxation of cervical vertebrae which may lead to neurologic deficits; septic arthritis of knees, elbows, wrists (staphylococcus most common)—19% mortality if not treated early

R/o:

- Osteoarthritis: improved after rest and worsens w activity; weight-bearing joints; distal interphalangeal (Heberden's nodes); proximal interphalangeal
- PMR (see pp 215–217)
- Gout (see pp 217–220)
- Pseudogout: common in knees, but may also be seen in the wrists, carpal joints; calcium pyrophosphate crystals in joint fluid
- Primary Sjögren's syndrome presents in elderly: milder; less positive ANA, fewer antibodies to SS-A, SS-B; more in RA
- Fibromyalgia: multiple tender points; disturbed sleep; no synovitis
- Scleroderma: may present w diffuse swelling of digits, but will also see skin changes and anti–Sci-70 antibodies; Raynaud's phenomenon
- SLE: 15% of pts present after age 50 yr; less female predominance in the elderly; milder course w fewer renal changes and more serositis and joint manifestations; rheumatoid factor occurs more frequently while hypocomplementemia and anti–double-stranded DNA antibodies occur less frequently in elderly SLE patients
- Polymyositis/dermatomyositis
- Carcinomatous polyarthritis: direct invasion of bones or joints by lung or breast malignancy; asymmetric; spares small joints; mild inflammatory joint fluid; xrays nl

Lab: Rheumatoid factor in 70% of pts, ESR >40 mm/h (elderly run high); mild normochromic, normocytic anemia

Xray: Periarticular osteopenia; periarticular soft tissue swelling; symmetric joint involvement; loss of cartilage; deformities (usually in late disease)

Rx:

Therapeutic (Nejm 1994;330:1368):

- ASA 650–1000 mg qid (elderly more susceptible to salicylism and possible development of pulmonary edema and high risk for gi irritation and bleeding); ASA + NSAIDs may decrease institutionalization rate (J Am Ger Soc 1996;44:216)

- Gold (toxic in elderly, causes diarrhea, rash, ulcers, nephropathy, marrow depression, colitis, so check CBC, UA, q 2 wk then q mo) 3 mg bid
- D-penicillamine 250 mg qd–tid (toxic in elderly; skin rash and taste abnormalities more common in elderly)
- Hydroxychloroquine 200 mg qd–bid (maculopathy more frequent in elderly)
- Azathioprine 50 mg qd–tid—beneficial effects within 2–6 mo
- Methotrexate 5–15 mg once a week (oral ulcers, liver abnormalities, marrow suppression, pneumonitis)
- Sulfasalazine 1–3 gm/d in divided doses (nausea and vomiting more common in the elderly), check lytes, BP, blood sugar, CBC, fecal occult blood test q 1–3 mo
- Steroid injections no more frequently than q 3 mo, use systemic steroids for short courses in conjunction w other agents; steroid side effects in 2–4 wk
- Obtain neck films of pts w long-standing RA and limited range of motion of neck to detect subluxation

Team Management: Physical and occupational therapy
- Acute episodes: avoid pillows under knees, prevents contractures
- Knee, ankle, wrist splints part of the day to stabilize painful joint while still allowing function
- Isometric maximal contraction of muscle groups in mid-joint range
- Raised soft heel protector for Achilles tendonitis
- Molded insoles to maintain longitudinal arch of shoe
- Hot soaks 20 min tid
- If other associated joints functioning, can consider joint replacement
- Swimming, water exercise if available
- Establish long-term relationships w occupational, physical therapists

POLYMYALGIA RHEUMATICA AND TEMPORAL ARTERITIS

J Am Ger Soc 1992;40:515

Cause: HLA-D4 genetic susceptibility; inappropriate immune response
Epidem: 0.1–1.0% of people over 70 yr; F/M = 2:1, white-black = 6:1
Pathophys: Medium and large arteries segmentally; smaller arteries may also be involved, eg, lung

Sx: May be sudden onset:
- Most w muscle pain which is relieved w activity
- Fever
- Jaw claudication
- Transient blindness or vision blurring (occlusion of ciliary artery causing infarction of optic nerve head or, more commonly, central retinal artery causing normal-appearing disk with the remainder of the retina pale w segmented vessels)
- Diplopia
- Headache usually unilateral
- Thickening of temporal artery

Also slower onset:
- W malaise
- Anorexia
- Weight loss
- Anemia

Less common sx of:
- Leg/arm claudication
- CHF
- Aortic arch syndrome
- Facial swelling
- Delirium/dementia
- Peripheral neuropathy

Si: Criteria for dx: shoulder or pelvic girdle pain or stiffness, morning stiffness >1-h duration, duration at least 4 wk, no muscle weakness on exam, no other collagen-vascular disease w elevated ESR, relief of symptoms within a few days of starting low-dose steroids, proximal muscle tenderness

Crs: Average duration 3 yr

Cmplc: Most PMR resolves uneventfully; 5% have synovitis in sternoclavicular joints; occasionally death (cerebrovascular infarct, MI, aortic aneurysm)

R/o RA, which responds to NSAIDs where PMR does not

Other causes of polymyalgia: SLE; dermatomyositis; periarteritis nodosa; neoplastic diseases, eg, carcinoma, multiple myeloma; Waldenström's macroglobulinemia; sarcoidosis, infective endocarditis, osteomalacia; HMG-CoA reductase inhibitors

Lab:

Chemistry: ESR >30 mm/h (80%–95%), often >100 mm/h; elevated plasma viscosity and CRP (80%–95%); normochromic, normocytic anemia (50%–80%); elevated globulin fraction in serum electrophoresis (50%); elevated alkaline liver function (50%); neg rheumatoid factor (85%); negative ANA (85%)

Invasive: Temporal artery bx: excise 3–5 cm because shorter segment may miss involved segment; if bx neg, still a 5%–10% chance that dx has been missed; bx rarely causes scalp necrosis, but more likely when both arteries are removed

Rx:

Therapeutic:

- PMR: 10–20 mg prednisone qd initially; then 5–10 mg reductions at monthly or 2-mo intervals, then reduced by 1-mg increments; may need to increase steroid dose w flare-ups which usually occur within the 1st year; 10%–25% of pts develop temporal arteritis as a flare
- Temporal arteritis: 40–80 mg prednisone in divided doses; vision loss: may need high-dose steroids, eg, 240 mg prednisone or 1000 mg iv bid × 5 d, ESR falls in 2 wk and is nl by 4 wk; then begin taper; reduce daily steroids by about 10% every 2 wk, will probably require 15–30 mg steroids for 2–5 yr w annual to semiannual attempts to taper meds; alternate-day steroid therapy not recommended; after corticosteroids discontinued, monitor pt for at least 6 mo, checking ESR
- Reduce cumulative doses of steroids w depot methylprednisolone acetate 120 mg im q 3 wk for 12 wk, or by using concurrent azathioprine or methotrexate (Abrams WB, ed, Merck manual of geriatrics, 1995)

HYPERURICEMIA AND GOUT

Ann IM 1979;90:812

Cause: Hyperuricemia defined as plasma urate >420 μmol/L (7.0 mg/dL); indication of increased total body urate due to overproduction and/or underexcretion of uric acid; plasma and extracellular fluid saturation with urate leads to crystal formation and deposition; uric acid is the final breakdown product of purine metabolism; two-thirds to three-fourths excreted in kidney and the rest is excreted in the small intestine

Epidem: More common in women

Pathophys: Gout—a group of disorders characterized by:
1. Hyperuricemia
2. Attacks of acute, monoarticular inflammatory arthritis
3. Tophaceous deposition of urate crystals in and around joints
4. Interstitial deposition of urate crystals in the renal parenchyma

Si: Extraordinarily painful joint, exquisitely sensitive to touch/pressure; patients don't tolerate any but gentle exam; may be subacute or chronic pain; tophi likely to occur in and around Heberden's nodes

Complc: R/o pseudogout calcium pyrophosphate deposition (more common in elderly, in larger joints, often following trauma, surgery, or ischemic heart disease); associated w hyperthyroidism; pos birefringent rhomboid crystals under polarized light; xray chondrocalcinosis in wrists, knees, pubis symphysis

Crs: Attacks less frequent in the elderly

Lab:
- Evaluation of hyperuricemia: >800 mg/24 h in urine indicates overproduction
- Aspiration of involved joint or tissue key to dx with demonstration of intracellular monourate crystals in synovial fluid, PMNLs, or tophaceous aggregates; needle-shaped crystals show strong neg birefringence

Rx:

> **Preventive:** Most individuals who are hyperuricemic never develop gout; therefore routine screening for asx hyperuricemia is not indicated; for diet, avoid high-purine foods (shellfish, wild game, organ meats); alcohol, dehydration can precipitate attack; if pt has diseases w increased cell breakdown, watch for increased production

> **Therapeutic:** Asx hyperuricemia: treatment is not beneficial or cost-effective except for chemotherapy pts (overproduction) who are at risk for acute uric acid nephropathy

> *Acute Gouty Arthritis*
> - NSAIDs: better tolerated than colchicine (former first-line treatment); indomethacin—most widely used in younger age groups but more toxicity in elderly; continue 3–4 d after all signs of inflammation have disappeared; use with caution in patients w PUD, heart failure, HT because of problems with salt retention; may precipitate hyperkalemia and renal insufficiency; anemia, check CBC early and during use

- Colchicine: can be useful if NSAIDs not tolerated; inhibits the release of leukocyte-derived crystal-induced chemotactic factor; oral doses of 0.6 tid, cannot be tolerated in up to 80% pts because of abdominal pain, diarrhea, and nausea; increased toxicity when given w other drugs that are P-450 enzyme inhibitors, eg, cimetidine, erythromycin, tolbutamine (Nejm 1996;334:445); can also be given iv but w significant toxicity risks; in pts with renal insufficiency, colchicine may produce a reversible neuromuscular toxicity that leads to a subacute myopathy, axonal neuropathy, and increased serum creatinine kinase
- Intra-articular injection of corticosteroids: use when pt cannot take po and when colchicine and NSAIDs are contraindicated or ineffective; po steroids (60–80 mg w quick taper), im steroids (methylprednisone acetate (Depo-Medrol) 50 mg), im ACTH can also be effective but unavailable at most pharmacies

Chronic Gout (patients with recurrent attacks, chronic sx, evidence of tophi, gouty arthritis, or nephrolithiasis):

- Biggest issue in elderly is toxicity of long-term med use for chronic gout; all use worth evaluating periodically; stop drugs if possible
- Before starting a urate-lowering agent, pt should be free of inflammation and have started colchicine for prophylaxis (0.6 mg tid is 90% effective in preventing further attacks); treatment goal is urate concentration <300 μmol/L (<5.0 mg/dL); diet modification plays a helpful role but pharmacotherapy is also effective; roles of hyperlipidemia, obesity, DM, HT, and ETOH abuse should be addressed
- Colchicine at 0.6 mg/d for long-term suppression if only sx is joint pain—low-risk regimen
- Allopurinol (for overproducers only): potent competitive inhibitor of xanthine oxidase; absorbed from the gi tract; half-life – 3 h; for pts with evidence of urate overproduction, nephrolithiasis, renal insufficiency (creatinine clearance <80 mL/min), tophaceous deposits, pts at risk for acute uric acid nephropathy; maximum reduction in urate seen at 2 wk; initiation may induce gout attack so concomitant colchicine is usually prescribed; minor side effects: skin rash, gi, diarrhea, headache; serious side effects: alopecia, fever, lymphadenopathy, bone marrow suppression, hepatic toxicity, interstitial nephritis, renal failure, hypersensitivity vasculitis; death can occur in pts with renal insufficiency

and pts taking diuretics; *drug interactions:* allopurinol prolongs the half-life of 6-mercaptopurine, cyclophosphamide, and azathioprine, all of which are degraded by xanthine oxidase; pts taking ampicillin or amoxicillin have a 3-fold increase in skin rashes; more toxic in the elderly, therefore reduce doses to 100 mg qod

• Uricosuric agents (for underexcretion, most common cause): decrease serum urate by inhibition of proximal tubule reabsorption; use carefully w renal monitoring in pts >60 yr old, creatinine clearance <80; most commonly used agents:

1. Probenicid 250 mg po bid up to 1.5 gm/d
2. Sulfinpyrazone 50 mg po bid (maintenance dose 300–400 mg po tid/qid)

CERVICAL AND LUMBAR STENOSIS (SPINAL STENOSIS)

Clin Ger Med 1994;10:557; JAMA 1995;274:1949

Cause: Congenital size of spinal canal and progression of degenerative spinal disease (soft and bony tissue) lead to vascular compromise of nerve roots (claudication sx) caused by a 50% reduction in one segment relative to normal segments above and below as seen on CT

Epidem:

Pathophys: Most common at L4/L5 or L3/L4 where there is disk degeneration leading to anterior, posterior disk height reduction and longitudinal ligament laxity and subluxation of facet joints; ligamentum flavum posteriorly hypertrophies in effort to keep segments from falling off each other, resulting in spinal stenosis

Sx: Cervical: upper extremity radiculopathy, loss bowel, bladder functions, lower extremity spasticity, pos Babinski, sensory changes

Lumbar: calf, leg, quad, hip pain after walking a discrete distance; back pain less common; lumbar spinal canal increases in size w flexion and decreases w extension; therefore standing, walking on flat surface, or downhill, which extends the spine, increase pain

Si: Neurologic exam usually neg w earliest sx but can progress to asymmetric ankle jerk, knee jerk; decreased quad, anterior tibial, extensor hallucis longus strength (check heel and toe walking, hip abduction); bicycle test (can bike further than can walk, for in sitting position lumbar spine is flexed, which opens up spinal canal and the foramen at each level); straight-leg raising neg; repeating exam after pt walks downhill may bring out subtle neurologic signs (Jama 1995;274:1949)

Cmplc: R/o:

- Acute and chronic disk pain increased by sitting forward; pts often roll to one side and sit up sideways; plantar flexion = L4, dorsiflexion and hip adductors = L5; clearer dermatome pain distribution; chronic disk herniation pain may closely mimic spinal stenosis pain
- Acute central disk: saddle anesthesia; sphincter tone loss (can be common finding in elderly); crossover leg pain (Bull Rheum Dis 1983;33:1)
- Peripheral vascular claudication: pulses absent
- Tumor or infection: rapidly increasing pain or dysfunction, night pain

Xray: LS spine film helpful; MRI

Rx:

Preventive: General conditioning, particularly walking

Therapeutic:

- Conservative: bicycling program, follow pt over long enough time to get careful reading on trend of sx before costly therapy; walker, wheelchair with exercise (NH patients)
- Acupuncture, acupressure, stress reduction, pain treatment programs (Semin Spine Surg 1994;6:156)
- Spinal manipulation not recommended (BMJ 1995;311:349; Ann IM 1992;117:590)
- Epidural steroids (Anesthesiology 1994;81:923)
- Surgical: posterior decompression helps calf pain mostly (2 wk–2 mo back to normal activities); fusion (4–6 mo back to normal activities); 85% of pts helped, 12% of pts no better, 3% of pts worse (J Neurosurg 1994;81:699; Spine 1992;17:1); no randomized trial has compared efficacy of surgical vs conservative rx (J Am Ger Soc 1996;44:285); rapid increase in surgical intervention w high regional variation suggests need for more research on pt selection (Wennberg J, Dartmouth Atlas of Health Care in the United States, Chicago: American Hospital Publishing, 1996)

PAGET'S DISEASE OF THE BONE

Clin Ger Med 1994;10:719

Cause: Autosomal dominant characteristics; 7 × greater risk if 1st-degree relative afflicted

Epidem: 2nd most common bone disease (after osteoporosis) affecting older population; although severe disease much less common

Pathophys: Localized increased rate of bone turnover and blood flow; pelvis, axial skeleton, skull, and weight-bearing bones affected most frequently; large increase in number and size of osteoclasts and increase in number of nucleoli; irregular resorption of bone produces "mosaic pattern"; reactive osteoblasts produce less organized "woven" bone

Sx: 5% experience pain, especially at night in warm bed secondary to vasodilation in vascular bone; fractures, hip arthritis; 1% develop osteosarcoma which presents w excruciating pain unrelieved by analgesics; when pt's skull affected, may become apathetic and lethargic (South Med J 1993;10:1097); mental status changes could result from shunting of blood from internal to external carotid system through anastomotic channels; bone compression of CNs II, V, VII, VIII produces monocular visual loss, atypical trigeminal neuralgia, facial paresis or paralysis, hearing loss; middle ear ossicles may be affected as well

Si:

- Deformities: anterior tibial bowing along lines of least resistance; anterolateral femoral bowing; weight of skull causes it to sink into spine, producing short neck and compression of cranial nerves at the base of the skull, spinal neuropathy, hydrocephalus from distortion of the sylvian aqueduct and obstruction of CSF
- Vertebrae: kyphosis, nerve entrapment, spinal stenosis, vascular steal syndrome which may be mistaken for direct cord compression (Aust NZ J Surg 1992;62:24)

Crs: Variable

Cmplc: Osteosarcomatous changes (Clin Orthop 1991;265:306); high-output CHF; heart block due to bundle calcifications; renal stones, especially w immobilization; r/o viral, traumatic causes of bone pain

Lab:

- Alkaline phosphatase reflects activity of the osteoblasts (Horm Metab Res 1991;23:559); be aware of commonness of minor alkaline phosphatase elevations in normal elderly—need elevations (1½–2× normal) to pursue dx

- Urinary hydroxyproline levels reflect activity of osteoclasts and bone resorption; both lab values used to monitor active disease and response to rx
- Urine and serum calcium nl unless suddenly immobilized; secondary hyperparathyroidism not uncommon

Xray: Trabecular and cortical bone irregularly thickened; sclerosis and deformity of periarticular bone; fissure fractures perpendicular to long axis of bone; inner and outer table of skull bones indistinguishable; thus entire thickness consists of spongiosa, producing "cotton wool" appearance; w osteosarcomas (most commonly in pelvis, femur, humerus) technetium uptake reduced and gallium uptake increased

Rx

Therapeutic:

- Treat asymptomatic Paget's disease of the skull or vertebrae; otherwise only rx disability, pain (not relieved by analgesics), increased bone deformity, frequent fractures, vertebral compression, rapid decline in hearing, high-output CHF
- Early intervention w CN decompression results in better prognosis
- Biphosphonates: etidronate 200–300 mg/d in frail elderly for 6 mo; alendronate (Fosamax): reduces the rate of bone turnover and decreases bone blood flow, newly formed bone is lamellar; effects long lasting and persist after treatment is stopped and more effective than etidronate and calcitonin (Nejm 1997;336:558) tiludronate (Sanofi) might be tolerated better than other biphosphonates (Med Let 1997;39:65)
- Calcitonin: 100 units qd for 3–6 mo followed by 50 units 3×/wk; urinary alkaline phosphatase and hydroxyproline should be halved in 3 mo; nausea from calcitonin self-limited and <10% of patients discontinue med; other side effects include flushing, diarrhea, and pain at injection site; human calcitonin has more side effects than salmon calcitonin; recrudescence when therapy discontinued even after a year of therapy
- Plicamycin: cytotoxic antibiotic reserved for nerve compression; 15–20 μg/kg over 5–10-d period; give w calcium and vit D
- Surgical hip replacement (J Bone Joint Surg Am 1987;69:760); total knee replacement (J Bone Joint Surg Am 1991;73:739)

LOW BACK PAIN

J Am Ger Soc 1993;41:167

Cause: Soft tissue trauma, including major and minor trauma, and overuse injuries; UTI; cancer; spontaneous vertebral compression fractures (osteoporosis)

Epidem: Very common in elderly; frequently chronic

Sx: Nonspecific limb sx (pseudoclaudication), loss of continence

Si: Lower extremity muscle strength, lower extremity muscle circumference, lower extremity reflexes, lower extremity sensory exam, straight-leg raising, sitting knee extension, palpate for lower abdominal masses; pelvic and rectal exam if pain severe or long-standing

Palpate point and general tenderness—spinous processes of lumbar vertebrae, iliolumbar ligaments, lumbar paravertebral muscles, sacroiliac joints, gluteal muscles; evaluate landmark asymmetries—leg length discrepancies, tibial tuberosities, iliac crest heights; pelvic compression—osteopathic maneuver to detect sacroiliac joint instability; pelvic roll—osteopathic maneuver to detect mobility of LS spine; standing and seated flexion; sacral motion

Complic: R/o fracture, spinal stenosis, infection, tumor, cauda equina syndrome

Lab: CBC, alkaline phosphatase, Ca^{2+}, PO_4^-, ESR, UA, serum immuno-electrophoresis later if suspect multiple myeloma

Xray: LS plain films can be useful if suspect fracture or neoplasm; prior film(s) always helpful for comparison; bone scan if suspect malignancy or osteomyelitis

Rx: Brief bed rest periods only (if at all); encourage brief walks; discourage sitting (particularly in auto) for any lengths of time; maintain regular f/u (frequency depends on pain); firm bed, lumbar pillow, abdominal muscle-strengthening exercises

Osteopathic:

Principles of Treatment:
- Use shorter, less frequent treatments
- Avoid thrust techniques in people with severe osteoporosis or osteoarthritis
- Re-establish motion as quickly as possible
- Use steady, gentle techniques

Specific manipulative treatments:
- Muscle and fascial stretching
- Muscle energy technique: improve muscle resting length by having pt actively engage the muscle group and then passively stretch it during relaxation
- Counterstrain: reduction of inappropriate neuromuscular reflexes by placing joint into a position of comfort for 90 sec
- Facilitated positional release
- Craniosacral technique: release of restriction of motion within cranial bones, spinal column, and sacrum and supporting fascia
- Soft tissue release: massage of muscle to improve fluid mobilization

Team Management: Establish physical therapy or osteopathic relationship early if musculoskeletal origin of pain

ADHESIVE CAPSULITIS OF SHOULDER
(BURSITIS, TENDONITIS)

Ger Rev Syllabus 1996; p. 237

Cause:
- Adhesive capsulitis: often times secondary to impingement syndromes

Epidem:

Pathophys:
- Adhesive capsulitis: contraction glenohumeral capsule

Si:
- Long head biceps tendonitis: arm motions w fixed flexed elbow, eg, screwing caps on jars; working overhead forcefully turns planter surface of hand upward against resistance with elbow fixed; tennis serve motion
- Rotator cuff tendonitis: 60–120 degrees extension with painful arc, pain at anterolateral aspect shoulder at greater tuberosity of humerus may lead to complication of subdeltoid bursitis, giving pain at tip acromion and over humeral head
- Subacromial bursitis: swelling, warm, tender
- Adhesive capsulitis: decreased movement of the shoulder

Table 10-1. Duration and Adverse Effects of NSAIDs

| | Half-life | | |
	Short	Intermediate	Long
Least side effects	Ibuprofen (Motrin)	Sulindac (Clinoril)	Nabumetone (Relafen)
Mid	Fenoprofen (Nalfon)	Naproxen (Naprosyn)	Piroxicam (Feldene)
	Indomethacin (Indocin)	Ketoprofen (Orudis)	
		Tolmetin (Tolectin)	
Most side effects	Meclofenamate (Meclomen)		

From BMJ 1996;312:1563.

Crs:
- Adhesive capsulitis: initial pain phase 2–4 mo, followed by limited shoulder mobility 4–8 mo, then gradual return to nl range of motion 6–12 mo (J Bone Joint Surg Am 1978;60:564)

Cmplc: Stage III after age 40: inflammation, permanent scarring, rotator cuff tendonitis tear, bone alterations, ruptured biceps

Xray:
- Adhesive capsulitis: nl xray, no degenerative bone loss
- Subacromial bursitis: calcific deposits on xray

Rx:

Therapeutic:
- Long head biceps tendonitis: rx bid w exercise; should improve in 3 wk; if not better in 6 mo, consider surgery
- Rotator cuff tendonitis exercises: pendulum, walk fingers up wall
- Heat before, ice after more strenuous exercise (when ready)
- Subacromial bursitis: 75% improve with steroid injections (Ann Rheum Dis 1984;43)
- Adhesive capsulitis: 6–12 mo—gradual return to nl w physical therapy; use analgesics and NSAIDs

NSAID use and Interactions (Table 10-1)
1. Antacids make NSAIDs more tolerable, but decrease absorption; gi toxicity reduced by misoprostol 100 µg qid (limited by diarrhea), assessment and possible treatment of *Helico-*

bacter pylori infection before commencing long-term course NSAIDs in pts w h/o recurrent PUD
2. With anticoagulation interactions; gi bleed risk; decrease anticoagulant to achieve same PT or PTT; ibuprofen (Motrin), tolmetin (Toletin), sulindac (Clinoril) have least gi adverse effects
3. Antirheumatic agents: watch wbc, platelets
4. Diuretics: adjustment may be necessary to maintain antihypertensive effects
5. Lithium: decreased clearance so monitor level 7 d after beginning NSAID, indomethacin (Indocin), piroxican (Feldene) in particular
6. Methotrexate: displacement from protein-binding site increases its toxicity
7. Oral hypoglycemics: displacement from binding leads to sulfonylurea toxicity, particularly with fenoprofen (Nalfon), naproxen (Naprosyn), naproxen sodium (Anaprox)
8. Phenytoin: naproxen and fenoprofen (Nalfon) will displace, leading to phenytoin toxicity
9. Probenecid: increases plasma levels of most NSAIDs—can reduce levels of some NSAIDs (ketoprofen, meclofenamate (Meclomen), indomethacin (Indocin))
10. Renal insufficiency relative contraindication, ASA alternative and can monitor w drug levels

11. Gastrointestinal Disorders

PEPTIC ULCER DISEASE

Surg Clin N Am 1994;74:93,113; Sci Am 1995;4(2):1; Jama 1996;275: 622

Cause: Smoking, aspirin, NSAIDs, *Helicobacter pylori* grows in mucus overlying antral gastric mucosa cells, and in 95% of pts w duodenal ulcers and 60%–75% of pts w gastric ulcers

Epidem: Mortality duodenal ulcer 2%–5%/100 000 elderly/yr; relapse 90% in 10 yr, quiescent after 10–15 yr; incidence increased in COPD, RA, cirrhosis, hyperparathyroidism

Sx: Duodenal ulcer: deep epigastric pain relieved by food or antacids; hunger experienced 2 h after meals; vomiting indicates ulcer within pyloric channel; melena from erosion at the base of the ulcer is an unusual complication, often asx in elderly

Cmplc: R/o:
1. Ischemic pain not relieved by food but may respond to vasodilator
2. Carcinoma: anorexia, nausea, weight loss
3. Acute cholecystitis: lancinating pain, fever, weight loss
4. Acute pancreatitis: nausea, emesis
5. Acute appendicitis
6. Other causes of upper gi bleeding (sources in order of decreasing prevalence): gastric ulcer, duodenal ulcer, gastric erosions, esophagitis, esophageal varices, neoplasm, Mallory-Weiss tears (J Am Ger Soc 1991;39:402)
7. GE reflux: rx w H_2 antagonist and prokinetic agent (metoclopramide (Reglan)) if sx's persist, and decrease dose by 50% in elderly

One-fifth of pts have complications:
- Bleeding ulcers
- Obstruction from edema or fibrosis in the region of the ulcer: distension or fullness before the meal is completed, >300 mL gastric contents 4 h after meal completed
- Perforation: highest mortality/morbidity in the elderly; severe progressive mid epigastric pain, later localizing to right lower abdomen if gastric contents spill along surface of right colon; can get posterior ulcer penetrating into pancreas causing acute pancreatitis, which rarely becomes recurrent or chronic

Lab: Endoscopy if gross upper gi bleed, no response to therapy, or multiple ulcers or gastric ulcer on previous exam, gastric ulcer

Basal and stimulated acid secretion when intractable to medical therapy, recurrent disease rapidly develops, gastric ulcer that might be caused by carcinoma (one-third of pts with ulcerated gastric carcinoma have achlorhydria after acid secretion stimulation whereas pts w benign disease have some acid secretion)

Breath urea test for *H. pylori* or rapid serologic tests (Nejm 1996; 333:984); antibody testing less specific than urease enzyme testing of bx specimen

Rx:

Therapeutic:
- Diets not effective, although pts may prefer to avoid foods that have troubled them; avoid caffeine; retrain from eating at night
- Antacids 1 and 3 h after meals and on retiring as good as H_2-receptor antagonists (Drugs 1994;47:305); MgOH—osmotic diarrhea; calcium-carbonate acid rebound; aluminum hypohospha temia—good for renal failure; alternating magnesium, aluminum, or calcium antacids avoids side effects
- H_2 receptors: rigorous separation of H_2 receptors and antacids probably not necessary; cimetidine available generically and 30%–50% less expensive; side effects: prolong half-life of phenytoin, theophylline, warfarin, β-blockers, lidocaine, diazepam, chlordiazepoxide because interact w hepatic P-450 microenzyme; cause mental confusion—big problem in hospital, since extensively used postop; after 2–3 mo rx for gastric ulcer, re-evaluate (UGI or endoscopy) to identify 5% who progress to gastric cancer; if sx of duodenal ulcer improve, no further study needed
- Sucralfate: 1 gm 1 h before meals 3×/d and hs; works for multiple gastric erosions as well; affects aluminum absorption (use w

caution in renal failure because of impaired excretion of aluminum); interferes w tetracycline absorption, constipation

- Anticholinergics: propantheline 30 min before meals; selective inhibitor gastric acid secretion
- Omeprazole: 20–40 mg; strongly inhibits hydrogen ion secretion by the gastric parietal cells; for resistant PUD, erosive gastritis; healing in 4 wk; interference w drugs metabolized by P-450 system; decrease in the acid-induced metabolism of ingested digoxin (Ann IM 1991;115:540); acute hepatic toxicity (Am J Gastroenterol 1992;87:523)
- Misoprostol: 200 μg qid; synthetic prostaglandin E_1 analogue for prevention of NSAID-induced gastric ulcers, also prevents duodenal ulcers
- *H. pylori* treatment: 2-wk course of amoxacillin 500 qid or clarithromycin 500 tid along w omeprazole 20 bid (Am J Gastroenterol 1994;89:39); triple-drug therapy w metronidazole 250 plus tetracycline 500 mg plus bismuth 2 tabs (all 3 doses qid w meals and evenings) results in >90% eradication—much less expensive alternative (Am Fam Phys 1995;52:1717)
- Sedation: oxazepam 10 mg tid
- Surgery: Billroth I or II for recurrent ulcers produces dumping syndrome in 10% of pts

DIVERTICULITIS

Surg Clin N Am 1994;74:293
See Table 11-1

Cause: Lack of dietary fiber

Epidem: >50% prevalence in persons over 70 yr

Pathophys: 90% in sigmoid colon because narrow caliber results in higher intraluminal pressure; found in R colon in the Asian population (Br J Surg 1971;58:902)

Sx: Pain 75% and hemorrhage 25%; abrupt, persistent L lower quadrant (sometimes R lower quadrant or suprapubic) colicky pain increasing in severity over time, exacerbated by meals, relieved by bowel movements; more often constipation than diarrhea or alternating; anorexia; vomiting; fever may be presenting complaint,

Table 11-1. Diarrhea

	Crohn's	Ulcerative Colitis	Diverticulitis	Mesenteric Ischemia	Villous Adenoma
Si/Sx/Lab	Blood/mucus/pus abdominal pain (postprandial)	Not as much bleeding as w younger pts	+/- Constipation, fever, leukocytosis, peritoneal sis; bleeding resolves spontaneously; be alert to presentation w few sx	↓ crampy postprandial pain; h/o decreased cardiac output, eg, Afib; may lead to diarrhea, distension, and 50% bleed within 24 h, and nausea and vomiting	Decreased K⁺; chronic diarrhea presentation
Xray/endoscopy/ complc	Ulcers or sigmoidoscopy; bx: transluminal granuloma; complc: obstruction, hemorrhage, perforation, fistula, malnutrition, weight loss large, arthritis, skin and oral lesions	Friable; avoid BE if fever; bleeding leads to toxic megacolon; 20% increase risk for colon cancer in 10 yr	Complc: obstruction, perforation, fistula, abscess, peritonitis from gram-neg and anaerobic organisms	BE thumbprinting (blue submucosal hemorrhage adjacent to pallor; heal 2 wk or 15% stricture; 20% persistent; 10% gangrene (w 90% mortality)	Colonoscopy
Rx	See p 233	See p 235	Surgical resection >2 episodes; early detection and rx w antibiotics important to prevent hospitalization	Rest bowel, parenteral fluids, NG tube, broad-spectrum antibiotics, surgery for gangrene or impending perforation, or if not resolved in 2-3 wk	Surgery

GASTROINTESTINAL DISORDERS

peritonitis; elderly may not have pain or fever, therefore serial exams important

Si: Distended abdomen, tympanic to percussion; bowel sounds diminished; localized tender mass; rebound tenderness locally; occult rectal bleeding

Crs: 3–10 d; recurrence rate 25% in first 5 yr

Cmplc: Perforation, fistula, abscess; urinary frequency, dysuria may suggest bladder involvement; most common cause of lower intestinal bleeding except angiodysplasia; w bleeding r/o angiodysplasia (R colon in two-thirds of pts, usually in the setting of previously undiagnosed asx disease, 70%–80% resolve spontaneously, 3%–5% require transfusions), colon cancer, ischemic bowel

Lab: Leukocytosis; white or red cells on UA if ureteral inflammation

Xray: Saw-toothed pattern and thickening of muscular wall of colon considered prediverticular condition; adynamic ileus, mechanical obstruction

Perform sigmoidoscopy early without vigorous bowel preparation and minimal air insufflation; wait weeks for full colonoscopy to r/o cancer proximal to rectosigmoid region

CT if suspect abscess

For continued bleeding: selective mesenteric arteriography to localize extravasation and distinguish from angiodysplasia, bleeding rate <1 mL/min technetium-tagged rbc scan w diverticular bleeding

Rx:

Therapeutic:
- Bowel rest w iv hydration
- Broad-spectrum antibiotics to cover gram-pos cocci, anaerobic and aerobic gram-neg organisms; tetracycline if no leukocytosis or fever
- β-Lactam antibiotic w activity against anaerobic and enteric gram-neg organisms and if no improvement, CT to r/o intra-abdominal abscess (pain may be lacking, may not have increased wbc, anemia, increased alkaline phosphatase, ESR may be only clues), fistula formation, surgical mortality 20%, try percutaneous drainage first
- Surgical consultation early
- Analgesics cautiously because they mask symptoms
- Diet can be advanced over few days to normal diet
- If severe, hemicolectomy indicated for spreading peritonitis; should be done in 2-stage procedure in the elderly unless can

Table 11-2. Findings on BE

Ulcerative Colitis	Crohn's
Loss of haustra; multiple 1-mm diameter "collar button" ulcers	"Rose thorn" ulcers w deep tracts; ileum involvement w skip lesions; "thumbprinting"; transmural involvement; fistulas

attain preoperative percutaneous drainage of isolated diverticular abscess

- For active bleeding, vasopressin for interarterial vasoconstriction, embolization; if pt exsanguinating, consider partial colectomy
- In select pts with early diverticulitis in NH or home w support, antibiotics and oral fluids w careful frequent evaluation appropriate

INFLAMMATORY BOWEL DISEASE (CROHN'S)

See Tables 11-1 to 11-3

Cause:

Epidem: Less common than ulcerative colitis, 16% of pts w Crohn's disease are >65 yr; bimodal population and involvement of different segments of the intestines in later years suggest different disease entities (Med Clin N Am 1994;78:1303)

Pathophys: Transmural; more likely to be distal part of small bowel, small bowel—narrowing ileal lumen

Table 11-3. Inflammatory Bowel Disease in the Elderly

Ulcerative Colitis	Crohn's
Slight male predominance	Female predominance
Severe initial attacks	Delays in dx
High mortality w severe attack	Mortality not increased
More frequent proctosigmoid	More colonic, less ileum involved
Lower relapse rate	Low postop recurrence rates
Good long-term prognosis	Good response med rx

Sx: Usually indolent; diarrhea persistent w large-bowel disease; less bleeding than ulcerative colitis; mucus, pus, and abdominal pain (postprandial) may resemble small-bowel obstruction if terminal ileum involved (Am Fam Phys monograph 1995;198:19)

Si: Aphthous ulcer in rectum

Crs: High (85%) postop recurrence (Med Clin N Am 1990;74;183)

Cmplc: Obstruction, perforation, fistula; malnutrition, 25-pound weight loss; arthritis; skin lesions; anal lesions; renal stones from calcium oxalate if terminal ileum involved

R/o:

- Cholelithiasis, cholecystitis
- PUD
- Mesenteric vascular insufficiency: pain disproportionate to belly tenderness; usually followed by bloody diarrhea within hours; treat w resection or re-establishment of arterial flow to involved bowel; chronic mesenteric ischemia presents w triad of postprandial pain, fear of eating, weight loss
- Tumors
- Amoebic colitis: associated w inanition, fatigue
- Irritable bowel: recurrent crampy pain, bloating, flatulence, diarrhea and constipation; pain associated w stress, relieved by passage of flatus or stool
- Bowel obstruction: periumbilical pain waxes and wanes q 10 min in lower bowel

Lab: Anemia secondary to iron deficiency, vit B_{12} metabolized in terminal ileum; folate deficiency from sulfasalazine inhibition of its absorption; mild leukocytosis >10 000/μL; can also see granulomas on bx in ulcerative colitis

Xray: Sigmoid ulceration on BE

Rx:

Team Management: In contrast to results in pts w ulcerative colitis, elemental diets and TPN w bowel rest improve symptoms, inflammatory sequelae, and nutritional status in pts w Crohn's (Nejm 1996;334:841)

ULCERATIVE COLITIS

Sci Am 1995;4(IV)
See Tables 11-1 to 11-3

Cause: Alteration in mucosal immune system
Epidem: 12% of pts are >60 yr; 3× more common than Crohn's
disease
Pathophys:
Sx: Tenesmus; presents more w diarrhea than bleeding in the elderly
Si:
Crs:

- Mild (60%, distal colon and rectum)
- Moderately severe (25%, >5 stools/d gross blood, cramping
  pain, intermittent temperature to 100.4°F, intermittent fatigue,
  increased sleep requirement)
- Severe (15%, extreme fatigue, weakness, prostration; distended
  abdomen, tympany, bowel sounds often absent); increased risk
  for colon cancer 20%/10-yr duration of Crohn's
- Extraintestinal manifestations: pyoderma gangrenosum, erythema
  nodosum, uveitis

Cmplc: Toxic megacolon 3%, perforation 3%, stricture 10%, severe
hemorrhage 4%, cancer 3% as high (40% in pts who acquired the
disease before the age of 15 yr) (Nejm 1990;323:1228); erythema
nodosum 3%, aphthous mouth ulcers 10%, iritis 5%, arthritic
large joints 5%, fatty liver 40%, pericholangitis 5%, cirrhosis 3%,
sclerosing cholangitis 2.5%

R/o bacterial gastroenteritis, ischemic colitis, diverticulitis, amebiasis,
Crohn's, irritable bowel
Lab: CBC, lytes, liver profile, blood cultures
Xray: Avoid BE if fever or tachycardia or increased rectal bleeding since
may cause toxic megacolon; friable sigmoid and rectum (grades
1–4 ranging from friability after swabbing to unprovoked bleeding before swabbing); small-bowel follow-through; pseudopolyps
(nodules of regenerative mucosa); aphthous ulcer rectum
Rx:

Preventive: Serial colonoscopies q yr w bx's q 10 cm after 8 yr of
the disease
Therapeutic:

- Antidiarrhea agents: diphenoxylate, loperamide, tincture of opium

- Sulfasalazine for remissions or mild sx: 0.5 gm bid × 2–4 d, then 0.5–1.5 gm qid (10% epigastric sx)
- Olsalazine (Gut 1994;35:1282), mesalamine for mild flares; corticosteroid enemas for mild to moderately active, 4 gm/60 mL (Gut 1992;33:947)
- Azathioprine 50 to 100 mg/d for several months; when bone marrow depression occurs, 3 d off drug will allow parameters to return to nl; ACTH 40 units iv q 12 h × 7–14 d for moderate to severe sx
- Add cyclosporine 4 mg/kg/day iv for fulminant colitis or toxic megacolon; response in 4 d
- Diet: watch for lactose intolerance
- Indications for proctocolectomy:
1. Failure of intensive drug therapy after 2–4 wk
2. Failure of toxic megacolon to improve after 4 d of intensive therapy
3. Cannot distinguish stricture from cancer
4. Severe extracolonic manifestations, ileal-rectal anastomosis or pouch (Ann Surg 1990;211:622)
- Antibiotics no help (Am J Gastroenterol 1994;89:43)

ISCHEMIC COLON

Med Clin N Am 1994;78:1303

Cause: Associated w artificial mitral valve, Afib, surgical bypass
Epidem: Most common cause of noninfectious colitis in the elderly
Pathophys: Mucosal, then serosal involvement; L colon (splenic flexure) better circulation
Sx: Abdominal pain (left-sided cramps in 75%), bleeding (50% within 24 h) distension, diarrhea, nausea, vomiting
Si: Decreased cardiac output
Crs: Bloody diarrhea, weight loss, decreased albumin, generally complete healing in 2 wk
Cmplc: Pseudo-obstruction, 15% strictures, 20% persistent ischemic colitis, 10% gangrene, 90% mortality
Lab:
Xray: BE: thumbprinting; sigmoidoscopy: focal hemorrhagic lesions, ischemic ulcerations (dark blue submucosal ulcerations adjacent to areas of palor

Rx:

> **Therapeutic:** Bowel rest, parenteral fluids; NG tube; broad-spectrum antibiotics; surgery if suspect gangrene or perforation impending or not resolved in a couple of weeks; of pseudo-obstruction: colonic decompression if cecal diameter >9 cm

ANGIODYSPLASIA (GI BLEEDING)

Clin Ger Med 1944;10:1

Cause:

Epidem: One of the most common etiologies of gi bleeding in the elderly; 25% associated w aortic stenosis (Am J Surg 1979;137:57)

Pathophys: Increased intraluminal pressure in the R colon leads to decreased mucosal blood flow and mesenteric ischemia leading to AV shunting in the submucosal layer of the bowel (Am Fam Phys 1985;32:93)

Sx:

Si: Bleeding from diverticular lesions (arterial source) more severe than from ectasias (venous source)

Crs: Usually stop spontaneously

Cmplc:

Xray: Colonoscopic findings: telangiectasias, surface erosions <5 mm cecum and ascending colon, tortuous veins

Rx:

> **Therapeutic:** Vasopressin, chemical embolization, electrocoagulation, laser, segmental resection, hemicolectomy

PANCREATITIS/CHOLECYSTITIS

Surg Clin N Am 1994;74:317

Cause:

- Pancreatitis: gallstones, meds (ethacrynic acid, corticosteroids, metronidazole, thiazide), metabolic (hypercalcemia, uremia), surgery, ERCP, sphincter of Odi dysfunction, tumors, ischemia, ?periampullary diverticula

Epidem:
- Pancreatitis: acute mortality rate 20% (Am J Surg 1986;152:638)

Pathophys: *Escherichia coli* and *Klebsiella* most common organisms in cholecystitis; anaerobic infections not uncommon

Sx:
- Cholecystitis: peritoneal signs are seen in fewer than half the pts and some pts have no abdominal tenderness; temperature frequently low grade, but may be toxic-appearing w pt disoriented and showing no abdominal signs; 40% of acutely ill pts have empyema, perforation, gangrene; 15% have subphrenic abscess or liver abscess; acalculous cholecystitis similar to acute calculous cholecystitis in presentation but most prevalent after surgery, trauma, repeated transfusions, burns, prolonged parenteral nutrition, cancer
- Pancreatitis: epigastric pain radiating to back; pt sits forward; tachycardia, nausea, vomiting, fever, ileus, shock; chronic pancreatitis presents w pain, nutritional deficiency w protein and fat malabsorption

Cmplc:
- Choledocholithiasis 10%–20% of time: presents w pain and jaundice 75% of time, pain 18% of time, jaundice 6% of time; endoscopic sphincterotomy if unfit for surgery; mortality rates for operative common duct exploration are 6%–12%, usually cardiac in nature
- Pancreatitis: left-sided effusions, localized parenchymal infiltrates (pancreatic effects on pulmonary surfactant) (Gastrointest Endosc Clin N Am 1990;19:433)
- Underlying adenocancer of the gallbladder: especially in women in 6th and 7th decades w gallstones
- R/o appendicitis

Lab:
- Cholecystitis: leukocytosis in two-thirds of pts
- Pancreatitis: elevation of enzymes not correlate w prognosis or severity of disease

Rx:
- Mortality from surgery for acute cholecystitis high (9.8%)
- ERCP, sphincterotomy for gallstone pancreatitis (Lancet 1988;2: 979)

ENTERAL FEEDING

Sci Am 1996;4(XIII):6; Nejm 1997;226:41

Indications: Pts w functional gi tract who are unable to sustain maintenance nutrition because of chronic anorexia or nausea, oropharyngeal obstruction, swallowing dysfunction

Type of Tube:
- NG tubes: 8–10Fr, soft, mercury-weighted tip
- Cyclic enteral overnight feeds 12–14 h for a minimum of 2 wk produces improvement in weight and cholesterol (Jama 1995;273:638)
- Gastrostomy tube if expect >6–8 wk; percutaneous placement requires minimal sedation (1% major complication rate)

Types of Formulas:
- Osmolite, Osmolite HN, Jevity, and Magna Cal; low in lactose; all contain some soy and corn, but also medium-chain triglycerides (MCTs) which are good for malabsorption; MCTs absorb directly into the portal system, not requiring action of bile salts or pancreatic enzymes; MCTs may be an ordered supplement to help with malabsorption

  Osmolite: 1.06 cal/mL; isotonic; 0.037 gm of protein/mL; USRDA daily requirements = 900 mL/d

  Osmolite HN (high nitrogen): 1.06 cal/mL; isotonic; 0.044 gm of protein/mL; 1400 mL/d to meet the USRDA; better for smaller people

  Jevity: equivalent to Osmolite HN plus fiber; hypoallergenic, good for diarrhea or constipation

  Magna Cal: high in calories, 2 cal/mL; hypertonic; 0.07 gm of protein/mL; good for people on fluid restriction

- Vivamax and Vivamax HN: made with crystalline protein (simple L-amino acids, easier to absorb); iso-osmolar
- Vital: a hyperosmotic, mixed-protein hydrolysate (eg, peptides) for pts on fluid restriction
- Criticare: mixed protein/peptide/amino acid; selected amino acids that are most necessary for those under increased stress
- Peptin: like Vital, but iso-osmolar, same as Vivamax
- Special products exist for hepatic and renal failure; others are pulmonary specific

Dose of Tube Feeds:

- Begin half strength, half the target volume; increase to three-fourths strength at the same infusion rate after 8 h; check residuals every 4 h and hold the tube feed for 4 h if the residual is greater than 50 mL; after 16 h, increase to full strength and keep the infusion rate the same; after 24 h, increase the rate to 75%–100% of the target rate; after 32 h use full strength and increase rate to 100% target rate; jejunal feeds continuous up to 125 mL/h
- Follow the sodium first few days; hypernatremia is common; give boluses of free water, about 100 mL every 6 h, periodically through the day

Indications for Peripheral Vein: For pts who are not hypermetabolic; supplement to enteral feeds

2.5–3.0-L limit restricts use by pts w renal or CHF; 286 kcal, 4.63 nitrogen/L: mix 500 mL 10% dextrose, 500 mL 5.5% amino acid solution plus fat emulsions; change catheter q 48 h to prevent thrombophlebitis; accurate weight, intake and output daily; lytes, BUN, glucose several times a week; liver function, calcium, phosphorus, magnesium, triglycerides q wk

HYPONATREMIA

See Table 11-4

Table 11-4. Hyponatremia (<135 mEq/L; <120 mEq/L = seizures)

	Decreased Serum Osm (<275)		NI Osm Hyperlipidemia	Increased Osm Hyperglycemia
	NI ECF	Decreased ECF	Hyperproteinemia	—
Increased ECF				
Urine Na <20/mEq/L CHF Cirrhosis	SIADH (CNS, lung, stress) Dilutional hyponatremia Urine Na >20/mEq/L Urine Osm >200 Morphine, tricyclics, nicotine, NSAIDs, sulfonylureas, hypo-natremia, adrenal insufficiency	Urine Na >20/mEq/L Renal Diuretic Addison's Dehydration	Hyperproteinemia	—
Rx: fluid restrict + furosemide; ?captopril	Water restrict; 0.9 or 3% saline + furosemide (increase Na 20 mEq/ L/48 h)	Replace fluid; rx underlying disorder	—	

ECF = extracellular fluid.

12. Dermatology

SKIN PROBLEMS (BENIGN AND MALIGNANT LESIONS)

Am J Med 1995;98:99S; J Am Acad Dermotol 1992;26:521; Nejm
1991;325:171; Am Fam Phys monograph 1995;193; Geriatrics 1993;
48:30

Cause:

Epidem: The incidence of skin cancers increases exponentially with age
and is thought to be related to UVB irradiation cumulated over a
life span

Pathophys: Changes of aging skin:

Epidermis:

- Flattening of dermal-epidermal junction leads to increased propensity to blister and erode following shear-type forces to the skin
- Decreased moisture content of the stratum corneum; decreased secretion from sweat glands; xerosis
- Decreased epidermal turnover: slowed wound healing; increased secondary infection following minor trauma, hyperproliferation disorders such as psoriasis tend to improve
- Melanocytes decrease by about 10% every decade after age of 30 yr, leading to depigmentation; melanin normally functions to absorb carcinogenic UV light
- Cell-mediated immune response decreased (Langerhans' cells or macrophages in the epidermis); more susceptibility to cutaneous tumors, but less potential for allergic contact sensitization

Dermis:

- The dermis decreases in density; relatively acellular, avascular, leading to poor insulation, pale skin, and hypo-hyperthermia; regression of subepidermal elastic fibers causes skin wrinkling; dermal clearance of foreign material decreased, prolonging contact dermatitis duration

Skin appendages:

- Sweat glands decreased causing dry skin, less body odor
- Pacinian and Meissner's corpuscles decrease by approximately two-thirds, predisposing elderly to trauma, burns, and decreased ability to perform fine hand maneuvers
- Subcutaneous tissue volume decreased within weight-bearing surfaces such as feet, causing calluses, corns, ulcerations, and chronic pain

ECZEMA

Appearance: Dry skin, fine fissuring, pruritic, lower legs, worsening in the wintertime

Rx: Of first importance, increase hydration by applying emollients and bath oils, particularly after bathing; avoid excess exposure to water; increase use of room humidifiers; only if severe or chronic, use steroid preparations:

- Classes III–VI (triamcinolone 0.025%–0.1%–0.5%), class II (fluocinonide (Lidex)), class I (betamethasone dipropionate (Diprolene) 0.05%, cream 0.05%), class VII (hydrocortisone, nonfluorinated 0.1%)
- Vehicle: lotion or gel for acute lesion (oozing, crusting, vesicles) to help drying; cream for subacute lesions (scales, patches); ointment for chronic lesions (dry skin, plaques, lichenification)

SEBORRHEIC DERMATITIS

Appearance: Greasy yellow scale w or w/o erythematous base on nasolabial folds, eyebrows, hairline, sideburns, posterior auricular, mid chest

Rx: Hydrocortisone 1.0%–2.5%

ROSACEA

Cause: Facial mite (possibly)

Rx: Dermodex w metronidazole 0.75% gel bid for 6–9 wk; rx pustules w doxycycline 100 mg po; telangectasias w electrodesiccation; rhinophyma w plastic surgery

PSORIASIS

Rx: Mild limited w topical corticosteroids, anthralin 1%–4%; recalcitrant cases w UV light, PUVA, topical vit D in limited doses because irritating; years of rx w UV light, methotrexate, cyclosporine, strong topical steroids may predispose pts to other health problems

SEBORRHEIC KERATOSIS

Appearance: Disseminated, pigmented, waxy, stuck on; may be very large or thickened
Crs: Benign
Rx: Electocautery, particularly for large lesions; liquid nitrogen may work
Look Alikes: Bowen's, superficial spreading melanoma

ACTINIC SENILE KERATOSIS

Appearance/Location: Multiple, red/brown, flat/raised, with adherent scale
Crs: Most common precancerous lesion in whites, but frequency of overall conversion debated; 12%—squamous cell (lip)
Rx: Liquid nitrogen—light 20-sec freeze/5-fluorouracil 2%–5% q d× 2–3 wk, may react w sun

BOWEN'S DERMATOSIS

Appearance: Two-thirds solitary, one-third multiple, sharply demarcated, scaly, flat or raised
Crs: Not sun-induced; good prognosis
Rx: Curettage; electrodesiccation; deep excision if hair follicle; topical fluorouracil bid several weeks to larger lesions; Moh's surgery and laser therapy are options also
Look Alikes: Eczema (palpable, thickened, red/brown w deepened skin lines), tinea, superficial basal cell, irritated seborrheic keratosis

KERATOACANTHOMA

Appearance: Common in elderly men, dome-shaped, flesh-colored smooth nodule with depressed center filled with keratin plug; sun-exposed areas; backs of hands, arms, central face

Crs: Rapid growth 2 wk, stationary, involution

Rx: Hard to distinguish from squamous, so excision, curettage, fulguration for lesions <2 cm

SQUAMOUS CELL

Cause: Sun, coal tar, creosote oil, paraffin oil exposures; xray-induced

Appearance/Location: Head/forearm/neck/back; firm erythematous nodule with indistinct margins

Crs: Metastasize unpredictably—lymph nodes; most convert to malignant from actinic keratosis; ulcer = aggressive

Rx: Electrosurgery; chemotherapy; Moh's surgery; surgery—wide excision or Moh's dependent on location; radiation

LEUKOPLAKIA

Appearance: White plaque mucous membranes; hypertrophic

Crs: Precancerous; 10%–17% develop into squamous cell carcinoma (floor of mouth, ventral surface of tongue) 1–20 yr after initial onset

Rx: Excisional bx, electrodesiccation, liquid nitrogen, topical fluorouracil, laser

Look Alikes: Vulvar atrophy; lichen sclerosis et atrophicus (extends beyond mucous membrane to skin; if doesn't respond to topical estrogen or corticosteroid, should bx, although potential for malignancy is small); candidiasis, 2nd syphilis

SCABIES

Appearance: 2–3 wk get first-time itching erythematous, papular eruption; excoriation, secondary infection; axillary, waist, inner thigh, back, arm, leg; burrows between fingers

Crs: Persists for decades untreated

Rx: Scrape skin parallel to surface of burrow deep enough to cause pin-point bleeding, use mineral oil and coverslip on slide to identify mite, egg, or fecal material; Kwell (lindane) 1% or Eurax (crotamiton) 10% or permethrin cream 5% × 12 h, reapply in 1 wk, itches for 2 wk; vacuum rugs, hot water wash, then heat dry clothes, treat close contacts

Look Alikes: Other bites (not in web spaces)

HERPES ZOSTER

Appearance: Tingling or pain 4–5 d, erythematous grouped vesicles/crust; occasionally nodules, papules; may affect eye (corneal ulceration); usually unilateral if on tip of nose; any dermatomes may be involved

Eye Findings:
1. Simplex—dendritic ulcers of cornea
2. Zoster—periphery of cornea with vascularization, ulceration, dendrites can happen—uncommon

Crs: Often extended course of many weeks to several months w "post-herpetic" pain; some communicability and best to avoid unnecessary exposure; NH staff require gloves if vesicles, crusting

Rx: If early, valacyclovir 1 gm tid × 7 d or famciclovir 750 mg tid × 7 d or acyclovir 800 mg 5×/d × 7–10 d; if established for >3 d, antivirals probably not helpful (and are expensive); if no contraindication to corticosteroids (DM, HT, glaucoma) prednisone 60 mg tapered over 21 d (Nejm 1996;335:32); uveitis: topical corticosteroids w ophthalmologic consult, atropine to dilate pupils; pain management often a longer problem, since may require codeine or other opioids; for extended courses, long-term lower-dose antivirals can be helpful

BULLOUS PEMPHIGOID

Nejm 1995;333:1475

Appearance: Sudden-onset urticarial plaques or intact tense blisters; flexural blisters, spreading rapidly; immunofluorescent studies: C_3 along basement membrane

Rx: Untreated lesions may become extensive and highly symptomatic, resulting in death; early administration of prednisone 1.0 mg/kg/d gives best response; 2nd rx: azathioprine, cyclophosphamide, cyclosporine, methotrexate, tetracycline, dapsone, sulfapyridine; pulsed corticosteroids, plasmapheresis, high-dose immune globulin

Look Alikes: Pemphigus vulgaris: no urticarial plaques; immunofluorescent studies: antibodies against intercellular cement

ONYCHOGRYPHOSIS

Appearance: Nails—patchy distal yellow discoloration; raised edge; more fragile, later thickening and curvature of nails due to chronic trauma; more extensive in pts w atherosclerosis, fungi, or chronic paronychial infection (usually secondary to candidal infection)

Crs: Chronic; rx expensive and of limited value in elderly w few long-term cures

Rx: VoSol or rubbing alcohol to affected nail fold results in evaporation of water in 10 min; if pseudomonas present, use gentamicin ointment or fluconazole; treat surrounding skin infections aggressively to improve comfort; nail cutting, grinding to reduce mass of nail important for foot comfort

MELANOMA

Appearance: Worrisome if asymmetric, irregular borders, >0.5 cm, multiple colors white, red, blue, black

Lab: Pathology of bx specimen: Clark levels:
I—limited to epidermis, no invasion
II—into but not filling papillary dermis, 95% 5-yr survival
III—filling papillary dermis
IV—reticular dermis
V—subcuticular fat, 5-yr survival 40%

Rx: Full excision primary lesion

ORAL CANCER

Epidem: Squamous 95%; risk factors: age, male, previous oral malignancy, tobacco, alcohol, exposure to sunlight (lip)

Crs: Prognosis without lymph node involvement: 50% 5-yr survival rate for tongue; 95% 5-yr survival rate for lip

Rx:

  Preventive: Quit smoking

  Therapeutic: High morbidity from surgical resection, irradiation, cytotoxic chemotherapy: disfigurement, speech impediment, salivary gland hypofunction, osteomyelitis

PRESSURE SORES

J Am Ger Soc 1995;43:919

Epidem: 50%–70% in pts older than age 70 in NH (J Am Ger Soc 1988;36:807); hospital prevalence 3%–11%, with highest in coronary care unit; on admission to NH 11%–35%, mortality risk for a NH patient with a pressure sore is 5–6× that of a NH patient without a pressure sore (J Am Ger Soc 1990;38:748)

Pathophys: When pressure exceeds 32 mmHg, capillary blood flow is halted; prolonged hypoperfusion leads to hypoxia, acidosis, hemorrhage into the interstitium (nonblanchable erythema), toxic cellular wastes, cell death, and tissue necrosis (Med Clin N Am 1989; 73:1511); pressure against the epidermis results in highest pressure nearest the bone, because pressure is more easily dissipated w deformation of the more superficial tissues

  Pressure, friction, shear, chronic exposure to water (Ped Derm 1994; 11:18), deficiencies in ascorbic acid, zinc, Fe (J Am Ger Soc 1993; 41:357)

Si: Table 12-1

Complc: Offending organisms in sepsis: *Proteus mirabilis, Escherichia coli, Pseudomonas aeruginosa, Klebsiella, Bacteroides fragilis;* recurrence of pressure ulcer within 2 yr of surgical primary wound closure (Adv Wound Care 1994;7:40)

Lab: ESR to r/o osteomyelitis (Jahnigen DW, 1995); serum albumin; CBC; serum glucose

Xray: Suspect osteomyelitis w elevated wbc, fever, and poor wound healing

Table 12-1. Staging of Pressure Sores

Stage I	Nonblanchable erythema of intact skin; early pressure sore may appear postoperatively as bruising
Stage II	Abrasion, opened blister, partial thickness involving epidermis and/or dermis
Stage III	Necrosis, undermining; full-thickness loss into the subcutaneous tissue
Stage IV	Sinus tracts, extension into the fascia, muscle, bone

Rx:

Preventive: Braden scale predictive value 64%–77% (Decubitus 1989;2:44) see page 48; and Norton scale predictive value 0%–37%; other similar scales (Am Fam Phys 1996;54(S):1519)

Address risk factors for pressure sores in all patients: lymphopenia, immobility, dry skin, decreased body weight (Jama 1995;273:865)

Nonblanchable erythema is very important early sign (address immediately); turn sequentially from back to left to right side q 2 h; avoid direct pressure on the greater trochanter and lateral malleolus by positioning back at a 30-degree angle to the bed w pillows between knees and lower legs and along back and arms to maintain optimal positioning (AHCPR Publc No. 92-0047, 5/92); reposition pts in chairs q 1 h; use trapezes, draw sheets; sitting on doughnut-type padding may cause ischemia (Ann IM 1986;105:337); education of multidisciplinary team decreased incidence of pressure sores by 63% (Arch IM 1988;148:2241)

Therapeutic:

1. Relieve pressure: mattresses and beds (list–J Am Ger Soc 1995;43:919); low-air-loss beds (Jama 1993;269:494); low-air-loss mattress cost-effective (J Gerontol 1995;141:6); air-fluidized beds for stages III–IV on two of the following areas: left hip, right hip, sacrum; or w recalcitrant wounds (J Am Ger Soc 1989;37:235)

2. Remove necrotic debris: chemical debridement w Granulex and Elase; dextramers may not be as effective

3. Control local infection: avoid systemic antibiotics unless there is an abscess or expanding cellulitis, then use clindamycin and floroquinolones; avoid topical antiseptics such as hydrogen peroxide, potassium hypochlorite (Dakin's solution), acetic acid, povidone-iodine (Betadine), may inhibit fibroblast growth (Clin

Ger Med 1992;8:835; J Trauma 1993;35:8); povidone-iodine may be more beneficial than saline dressings for short periods of time, eg, 4–5 d for purulent, odoriferous wounds (Postgrad Med J 1993;69:S97), 1:100 strength of povidone-iodine not harmful to wounds (Jahnigen DW, 1995); MRSA-infected wound: topical mupirocin (Bactroban) (Jahnigen DW, 1995); malodorous pressure sores: metronidazole gel (Am Fam Phys 1996;54(S):1519)

4. Protect healthy tissue: stages II and III w little exudate; use petroleum gauze, or semipermeable or occlusive dressing q 2–3 d

5. Promote granulation: moist environment hastens healing w increased migration of fibroblasts and growth factor; hydrocolloid dressing q 3–5 d for stages III and IV, better than wet to dry, watch for infection; deep wound packing w space-occupying (eg, calcium alginates) or salt-impregnated dressings (Mesalt) for stages III and IV (J Am Ger Soc 1995;43:919)

6. General condition: high-protein diet (24% protein) enhances wound healing (J Am Ger Soc 1993;41:357); ascorbic acid 500 mg bid (J Gen IM 1991;6:81); zinc 200–600 mg qd (Ann IM 1986;105:342)

Future treatment options: fibroblast growth factor (J Clin Invest 1993;92:2841), hyperbaric oxygen (Jama 1990;263:2216; Nejm 1996;334:1642)

13. Ethics

Clin Ger Med 1994;10:403; Arch IM 1995;155:502

COMPETENCY

See Tables 13-1, 13-2

"Informed consent" depends on competency, a legal definition; pt must demonstrate:

1. Ability to evidence a choice about treatment
2. Capacity to have factual understanding of the information that the average pt would consider material to making the health care decision in question
3. The ability to rationally manipulate information
4. The capacity to appreciate the nature of the specific situation (Am J Psychiatry 1977;134:3)

Mini-Mental State Exam (MMSE) not good for predicting competency, scores <7 incompetent, score 27 = competent, scores 7–27 not helpful (Folstein M, Bar Harbor, ME, 6/96); decision making capacity in elderly does not compare well to MMSE and should be assessed by direct methods (J Am Ger Soc 1990;38:1097; Am J Psychiatry 1977; 134:3); autonomy assumes that persons possess the capacity to decide, to carry out decisions, and to manage and be accountable for the consequences of their decisions (J Am Ger Soc 1995;43:1437)

ETHICS

Table 13-1. Competency Profile

Name:	SS#:		Date:	
Decision to be made:				
Criterion		Independent	With Assistance	Unable
1. Receives information				
2. Recognizes relevant information as information				
3. Remembers information				
4. Relates situation to oneself, values, and circumstances				
5. Reasons about alternatives				
6. Ranks alternatives in order of preference				
7. Resolves situations (dilemmas)				
8. Resigns self to the decision				
9. Recounts one's decision-making process				
10. Organizes effort to implement the decision				

From Nurs Home Med 1996;4:49A.

Table 13-2. Mnemonic for Evaluating Competency

"C"—consistent	Consistent on serial Mini Mental State Exam (MMSE); consistent decision on serial questioning; and consistent w life values
"O"—other alternatives to therapy	Understands other care alternatives, which, in turn, requires ability to understand factual material and manipulate information rationally
"M"—malleable	Physician must remain malleable; pts and families change their minds about end-of-life decisions in different settings and decisions should be reviewed w a change of setting
"P"—particulars	Pt must be able to appreciate the nature of the particular situation; physician must be particular about what pt is competent to do, eg, can decide health care but not run a household; degree of competence (supramaximal, full, limited) may differ depending on the domain (civil, personal, financial, health care) (Nurs Home Med 1996;4:81); least restrictive guardianship is the goal (partial capacity)

ADVANCE DIRECTIVES

Provide answers to the following treatment decisions:
1. Cardiac arrest
2. Acute, reversible, life-threatening event
3. Acute, nonreversible, life-threatening event
4. Nutrition
5. Routine blood work (J Am Ger Soc 1991;39:396,1221)

Directives completed at higher rates w physician-directed intervention (Arch IM 1994;154:2321); prehospital code status can be effectively made in the NH setting; have no effect on the short term but decrease use of hospital in the last months of life (J Am Ger Soc 1995;43:113)

Pts overemphasize benefit of CPR (J Gen IM 1993;8:295), but prognostic information influences decisions and most elderly do not want CPR (Nejm 1994;4:330,545); 14% of elderly will change opinion based on more information (Jama 1995;274: 1775)

Medical futility: physiologic intervention no plausible effect on disease;

quantitative: extremely unlikely to have effect on disease; qualitative: not improve, possible diminished quality of life

APACHE (Acute Physiology and Chronic Health Evaluation) predictors of mortality depend on severity of illness and not age; age alone does not predict survival (J Am Ger Soc 1995;43:520,1131; Am J Emerg Med 1995;13:389; Jama 1990;264:2109); decreased survival in hospitalized pts >70 yr old probably due to underlying medical problems; predictors of poor outcome following CPR: hct <35, creatinine >1.5, BUN >65, albumin <2.7 gm/dL (Ann IM 1989;7:199; J Am Ger Soc 1990;38:1057); success rate of CPR in elderly >70 yr old so low not worth it? (Ann IM 1989;111:193,199; Arch IM 1993;153:1293); poor outcome in NH facilities (J Am Ger Soc 1993;41:163,384)

Life values and resuscitation preferences are related; therefore important to discuss (J Am Ger Soc 1996;44:958)

Nutrition: Food and hydration are seen as basic human necessities; until the late 1970s providing artificial nutrition was not possible in most situations—just because we can provide it, should we? (Nejm 1984;311:402)

Basic human need vs extraordinary medical intervention (Clin Ger Med 1994;10:475); survey of NG tube feeds in elderly pts in a community hospital found that 53% of the time restraints were needed, and 24 of 29 pts were judged to be incompetent (Clin Ger Med 1994;10:475; Arch IM 1989;149:1937)

States have various statutes regarding when tube feeding can be stopped or not started (Clin Ger Med 1994;10:475)

Does starvation/dehydration cause pain and suffering?—complete starvation associated with euphoria and analgesia (J Gen IM 1993;8:220; Clin Ger Med 1994;10:475)

SUBSTITUTED JUDGMENT

Competent pt can leave advance directives (a living will, or durable power of attorney for health care); cannot infer CPR decision on basis of pt having a "living will" (Arch IM 1995;155:171)

Majority directives to carry out CPR are made by pts; the majority of DNR orders are made by families (Arch IM 1992;152:561; Jama

1985;253:2236); physicians and families are not good at predicting pt preferences (Arch Fam Med 1994;3:1057)

Long-term care residents at NH do not have long-term survival from CPR (J Am Ger Med 1993;41:163); modifications needed since poor survival in NH patients w unwitnessed arrest or asystole, electrical mechanical dissociation (J Am Ger Soc 1995;43:520); NH medical directors are more likely to support withholding rx in terminally ill pts, but are generally not in favor of mandatory DNR orders (J Am Ger Med 1995;43:1131; J Am Board Fam Pract 1993;6:91; Ann Emerg Med 1994;23:997)

If no appropriate surrogate can be found, then group of individuals who care for the pt may determine treatment (multidisciplinary health care team) according to American Geriatric Society (AGS) ethics committee position 3 (J Am Ger Soc 1996;44:986)

REFUSAL OF TREATMENT

Competent Patients: Have the right to refuse rx; rx against pt's wishes can be construed as assault and battery and has been prosecuted as such (Clin Ger Med 1994;10:475)

Incapacitated Patients: Rigid criteria such as permanent unconsciousness or poorly defined categories such as terminal condition inadequate alone to determine whether surrogate should have authority to refuse life-sustaining rx for pt because often substantial uncertainty about prognosis and most pt preferences are based on projected quality, not quantity, of life (AGS ethics committee position 8–J Am Ger Soc 1996;44:986)

Physician-Assisted Suicide (Euthanasia): More ethical solution might be rx of pain, especially in dying patients, and compassionate care; pts unduly influenced by physical suffering, impairment, abandonment, financial bankruptcy (J Am Ger Soc 1995;43:553); treatment of mild-to-moderate depression does not necessarily result in increased desire for life-sustaining measures (J Gerontol 1994;49: M15)

Withdrawing of Therapy: Not obligated to continue a therapy that is not accomplishing any of the predefined goals of therapy if the following conditions apply:

- Pt has irreversible loss of cognitive function
- No goal other than sustaining organic life is accomplished by therapy
- No other goals of therapy can be achieved
- Pt has not previously expressed preferences about being sustained in organic life (Clin Ger Med 1994;10:475); position supported by AMA council on ethical and judicial affairs

Withholding treatment vs withdrawing treatment—morally equivalent? no (J Am Ger Soc 1995;43:716,696) vs yes (President's Commission for the Study of Ethical Problems in Biomedical and Behavioral Research, US Government Printing Office, 1983)

Truth Telling (eg, Alzheimer's): When patient's decision making capacity and ability to cope w medical information is impaired enough to warrant withholding information vs withholding information that deprives patient of opportunity to act on important medical and nonmedical (financial planning) life decisions

Index